Fourth Edition

DRUG CALCULATIONS FOR NURSES

A STEP-BY-STEP APPROACH

Fourth Edition

DRUG CALCULATIONS FOR NURSES

A STEP-BY-STEP APPROACH

ROBERT LAPHAM

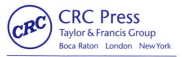

CRC Press
Taylor & Francis Group
Boca Raton London New York

CRC Press is an imprint of the
Taylor & Francis Group, an **informa** business

CRC Press
Taylor & Francis Group
6000 Broken Sound Parkway NW, Suite 300
Boca Raton, FL 33487-2742

© 2015 by Taylor & Francis Group, LLC
CRC Press is an imprint of Taylor & Francis Group, an Informa business

No claim to original U.S. Government works

Printed on acid-free paper
Version Date: 20150417

International Standard Book Number-13: 978-1-4822-4845-6 (Paperback)

Visit the Taylor & Francis Web site at
http://www.taylorandfrancis.com

and the CRC Press Web site at
http://www.crcpress.com

Do not worry about your difficulties in Mathematics. I can assure you mine are still greater.

Albert Einstein (1879–1955)

German-American physicist who developed the special and general theories of relativity

Contents

Preface

Drug treatments given to patients in hospital are becoming increasingly more complex. Sometimes, these treatment regimes involve potent and, at times, new and novel drugs. Many of these drugs are toxic or possibly fatal if administered incorrectly or in overdose. It is therefore very important to be able to carry out drug calculations correctly so as not to put the patient at risk.

In current nursing practice, the need to calculate drug dosages is not uncommon. These calculations have to be performed competently and accurately to ensure that the nurse – and more importantly the patient – is not put at risk. This book provides an aid to the basics of mathematics and drug calculations. It is intended to be of use to all nurses of all grades and specialities, and to be a handy reference for use on the ward.

The concept of this book arose from nurses themselves; a frequently asked question was: 'Can you help me with drug calculations?' Consequently, a small booklet was written to help nurses with their drug calculations, particularly those studying for their IV certificate. This was very well received, and copies were being reproduced from the originals, indicating the need for such help, and for a book like this.

The book's content was determined by means of a questionnaire sent to nurses, asking them what they would like to see featured in a drug calculations book. As a result, this book was written with the aim to cover the topics that nurses would like to see.

Although the book was primarily written with nurses in mind, it can also be used by anyone who uses drug calculations in their work. Some topics have been dealt with in greater detail for this reason (e.g. moles and millimoles). Therefore this book can be used by anyone who wishes to improve their skills in drug calculations, and it can also be used as a refresher course.

How to use this book

This book is designed to be used for self-study. Before you start, you should attempt the pre-test to assess your current ability in carrying out drug calculations. After completing the book, repeat the test and compare the two scores to see if you have made any improvement.

To attain maximum benefit from the book, start at the beginning and work through one chapter at a time, as subsequent chapters increase in difficulty. You should understand each chapter fully and be able to answer the problems confidently before moving on to the next chapter.

Alternatively, if you wish to quickly skip through any chapter, you can refer to the Key Points found at the beginning of each chapter.

CASE REPORTS

During the period 1991 to 2002, the journal *Pharmacy in Practice* highlighted various medication errors. These have been used throughout the book to illustrate various learning points.

ESTIMATIONS

It is good practice to estimate answers to drug calculations. Throughout the book, for all worked examples and answers to problems, estimations will be given before calculating the answers. Estimations are usually manipulations of numbers, and for simple calculations, most of the answers can be obtained by number manipulation. There are various means to estimate answers and by following those given in the book, readers will be able to see some of the techniques used, and hopefully develop their own.

ONLINE PRACTICE QUESTIONS

New to this edition is an online test bank featuring hundreds of practice questions. Test yourself, track your progress and refer back to the book to address your areas of weakness. Please go to www.drugcalcsnurses.co.uk to register.

Drug calculation questions are a major concern for most healthcare professionals, including nurses and those teaching them. There are numerous articles highlighting the poor performance of various healthcare professionals.

The vast majority of calculations are likely to be relatively straightforward, and you will probably need to perform complex calculations only infrequently. But it is obvious that people are struggling with basic calculations.

It is difficult to explain why people find maths difficult, but the best way to overcome this is to try and make maths easy to understand by going back to first principles. The aim is not to demean or offend anyone, but to remind and explain the basics. Maths is just another language that tells us how we measure and estimate, and these are the two key words. It is vital, however, that any person performing calculations using any method, formula or calculator can understand and explain how the final dose is actually arrived at through the calculation.

NUMERACY

Numeracy is used for a range of healthcare activities, such as measuring height and body weight, drug administration and for managerial tasks such as budgeting (Hutton 2009). Poor numeracy among healthcare staff is not new. It has always been a concern and is regularly raised in the media. Recently (May 2014) a trust chief executive quoted a failure rate of 50 to 80 per cent when testing nursing job applicants' literacy and numeracy skills (Lintern 2014).

In nursing and midwifery, the Nursing and Midwifery Council (NMC) has introduced several measures to improve the numeracy skills of nurses and midwives by introducing the concept of Essential Skills Clusters – ESCs (NMC 07/2007). Since 2008, applicants for pre-registration programmes must be able to manipulate numbers as applied to volume, weight and length (including addition, subtraction, division, multiplication and use of decimals, fractions and percentages) and be able to use a calculator (Axe 2011, NMC 03/2008).

Why do nurses regularly perform badly in numeracy tests? McMullan, Jones and Lea (2010) provided some suggestions: individuals who are anxious about performing numeracy may be drawn to people-oriented and caring careers such as those in healthcare. They also suggested an over-reliance on calculators and no practice in mental arithmetic in secondary schools as contributing factors.

The ESCs (NMC 07/2007) require the standard of a 100% pass mark for numerical assessment for nursing students graduating to registration. Young, Weeks and Hutton (2013) produced a list of numeracy skills (linked to the NMC ESCs) and where they are needed in nursing practice:

NUMERACY SKILL	EXAMPLE
Estimation	• All medication dosages
	• IV infusion rate calculations
Addition	• Fluid balance
	• Addition of doses of varying strengths (tablets, capsules, suspensions)
Subtraction	• Fluid balance
Multiplication	• Conversion of units
	• IV infusion rate calculations
Division	• Conversion of units
	• IV infusion rate calculations
Fractions	• Drip rate calculations
	• Enteral feeding
	• Conversion to SI units
Decimals	• Conversion of units
	• IV infusion rate calculations
SI Units	• Prescriptions
	• Haematology and biochemistry blood results
	• Patients' weight measurement and conversion
Conversion of units	• Paediatric dosages
	• Translation to imperial measures for patients/ relatives (e.g. birth weight)
Understanding percentages	• Distinguish between percentage expressions (e.g. 5% dextrose, grams/100 mL, 98% oxygen saturation, 2% management cuts)
Ratio	• Preparation of solutions
	• Medications dosage calculation
Use of formulae	• Dosage calculations
	• IV infusion rate calculations
	• Body surface area (BSA) estimation
	• Body mass index (BMI) calculation
Use of tables	• Conversion tables (Imperial/SI units)
	• BMI tables
Use of charts/graphs	• Temperature charts
	• Growth charts
	• Prescription charts
Appreciation of statistics	• Evidence-based practice

Continued

NUMERACY SKILL	EXAMPLE
Budgeting	• Stock control
Basic bookkeeping	• Helping clients with managing their money
Measurement	• Fluid balance
	• Vital signs
	• Preparing/drawing-up and dispensing medicines
Negative numbers	• Fluid balance
	• Ophthalmics
Recognition of indices	• Blood results (e.g. WBC 4.0×10^9/L)

References

Axe S. Numeracy and nurse prescribing: do the standards achieve their aim? *Nurse Education in Practice* 2011; 11(5): 285–287.

Hutton M. Numeracy and drug calculations in practice. *Primary Health Care* 2009; 19(5): 40–45.

Lintern S. Concern as nurses fail drug numeracy testing. *Health Service Journal* 2014; May 23: 13.

McMullan M, Jones R, Lea S. Patient safety: numerical skills and drug calculation abilities of nursing students and Registered Nurses. *Journal of Advanced Nursing* 2010; 66(4): 891–899.

NMC Circular 07/2007: Introduction of Essential Skills Clusters for Pre-Registration Nursing Programmes. Nursing and Midwifery Council, London.

NMC Circular 03/2008: The Evidence of Literacy and Numeracy Required for Entry to Pre-Registration Nursing Programmes. Nursing and Midwifery Council, London.

Young S, Weeks KW and Hutton BM. Safety in numbers 1: essential numerical and scientific principles underpinning medication dose calculation. *Nurse Education in Practice* 2012; 13(2): e11–e22.

To obtain the maximum benefit from this book, it is a good idea to attempt the pre-test before you start working through the chapters. The aim of this pre-test is to assess your ability at various calculations.

The pre-test is divided into several chapters that correspond to each chapter in the book, and the questions reflect the topics covered by each chapter. You don't have to attempt every chapter, only the ones that you feel are relevant to you. Answering the questions will help you identify particular calculations you have difficulty with.

You can use calculators or anything else you find useful to answer the questions, but it is best to complete the pre-test on your own, as it is *your* ability that is being assessed and not someone else's.

Don't worry if you can't answer all of the questions. The aim of the pre-test is to help you to identify areas of weakness. Again, you don't have to complete every section, just the ones you want to test your ability on.

Once you have completed the pre-test and checked your answers, you can the start using the book. Concentrate particularly on the areas you were weak on, and if necessary, miss out the chapters you were confident with.

It is up to you as to how you use this book, but the pre-test should help you to identify areas you need to concentrate on.

The pre-test consists of 50 questions and covers all the topics and types of questions in the book. Mark your score out of 50 and then double it to find the percentage.

BASICS

This section tests your ability on basic principles such as multiplication, division, fractions, decimals, powers and using calculators before you start any drug calculations.

Long multiplication

Solve the following:

1 678×465
2 308×1.28

Long division

Solve the following:

3 $3143 \div 28$
4 $37.5 \div 1.25$

Fractions

Solve the following, leaving your answer as a fraction:

5 $\dfrac{5}{9} \times \dfrac{3}{7}$

6 $\dfrac{3}{4} \times \dfrac{12}{16}$

7 $\dfrac{3}{4} \div \dfrac{9}{16}$

8 $\dfrac{5}{6} \div \dfrac{3}{8}$

Convert to a decimal (give answers to two decimal places):

9 $\dfrac{2}{5}$

10 $\dfrac{9}{16}$

Decimals

Solve the following:

11 25×0.45
12 $5 \div 0.2$
13 0.8×100
14 $64 \div 1,000$

Convert the following to a fraction:

15   1.2
16   0.375

Roman numerals

Write the following as ordinary numbers:

17   VII
18   IX

Powers

Convert the following to a proper number:

19 3×10^4

Convert the following number to a power of 10:

20   5,000,000

PER CENT AND PERCENTAGES

This section is designed to see if you understand the concept of per cent and percentages.

21 How much is 28% of 250 g?
22 What percentage is 160 g of 400 g?

UNITS AND EQUIVALENCES

This section is designed to test your knowledge on units normally used in clinical medicine, and how to convert from one unit to another. It is important that you can convert units easily, as this is the basis for most drug calculations.

Convert the following.

Units of weight

23 0.0625 milligrams (mg) to micrograms (mcg)
24 600 grams (g) to kilograms (kg)
25 50 nanograms (ng) to micrograms (mcg)

Units of volume

26 0.15 litres (L) to millilitres (mL)

Units of amount of substance

Usually describes the amount of electrolytes, as in an infusion (see the discussion in Chapter 4 on moles and millimoles for a full explanation).

27 0.36 moles (mol) to millimoles (mmol)

DRUG STRENGTHS OR CONCENTRATIONS

This section is designed to see if you understand the various ways in which drug strengths can be expressed.

Percentage concentration

28 How much sodium (in grams) is there in a 500 mL infusion of sodium chloride 0.9%?

mg/mL concentrations

29 You have a 5 mL ampoule of dopexamine 1%. How many milligrams of dopexamine is there in a 5 mL ampoule?

'I in …' concentrations or ratio strengths

30 You have a 10 mL ampoule of adrenaline/epinephrine 1 in 10,000. How much adrenaline/epinephrine – in milligrams – does the ampoule contain?

Parts per million (ppm) strengths

31 If drinking water contains 0.7 ppm of fluoride, how much fluoride (in milligrams) would be present in 1 litre of water?

DOSAGE CALCULATIONS

These are the types of calculations you will be doing every day on the ward. They include dosages based on patient parameters and paediatric calculations.

Calculating the number of tablets or capsules required

The strength of the tablets or capsules you have available does not always correspond to the dose required. Therefore you have to calculate the number of tablets or capsules needed.

32 The dose prescribed is furosemide 120 mg. You have 40 mg tablets available. How many tablets do you need?

Drug dosage

Sometimes the dose is given on a body weight basis or in terms of body surface area. The following tests your ability at calculating doses on these parameters.

Work out the dose required for the following:

33 Dose = 0.5 mg/kg   Weight = 64 kg
34 Dose = 3 mcg/kg/min   Weight = 73 kg
35 Dose = 1.5 mg/m^2 Surface area = 1.55 m^2 (give
                                answer to 3 decimal places)

Calculating dosages

Calculate how much you need for the following dosages:

36 You have aminophylline injection 250 mg in 10 mL.
     Amount required = 350 mg
37 You have digoxin injection 500 mcg/2 mL.
     Amount required = 0.75 mg
38 You have morphine sulphate elixir 10 mg in 5 mL.
     Amount required = 15 mg
39 You have gentamicin injection 40 mg/mL, 2 mL ampoules.
     Amount required = 4 mg/kg for a 74 kg patient; how many ampoules will you need?

Paediatric calculations

40 You need to give trimethoprim to a child weighing 22.5 kg at a dose of 4 mg/kg twice a day.
Trimethoprim suspension comes as a 50 mg in 5 mL suspension.
How much do you need for each dose?

Other factors to take into account are: displacement volumes for antibiotic injections.

41 You need to give benzylpenicillin at a dose of 200 mg to a 6-month-old baby. The displacement volume for bemzylpenicillin is 0.4 mL per 600 mg vial.
How much water for injections do you need to add to ensure a strength of 600 mg per 5 mL?

Prescribing

42 You want to prescribe lactulose 15 mL BD for 28 days. Lactulose is available as 500 mL bottles; how many bottles should be prescribed to ensure at least 28 days of treatment?

43 You want to prescribe ibuprofen 400 mg TDS for 28 days. Each 28 tablet pack of 400 mg tablets costs £1.12. How much will it cost to prescribe treatment for 28 days?

INFUSION RATE CALCULATIONS

This section tests your knowledge of various infusion rate calculations. It is designed to see if you know the different drop factors for different giving sets and fluids, and if you are able to convert volumes to drops and vice versa.

Calculation of drip rates

44 What is the rate required to give 500 mL of sodium chloride 0.9% infusion over 6 hours using a standard giving set?

45 What is the rate required to give 1 unit of blood (500 mL) over 8 hours using a standard giving set?

Conversion of dosages to mL/hour

Sometimes it may be necessary to convert a dose (mg/min) to an infusion rate (mL/hour).

46 You have an infusion of dopamine 800 mg in 500 mL. The dose required is 2 mcg/kg/min for a patient weighing 60 kg.
What is the rate in mL/hour?

47 You are asked to give 500 mL of doxapram 0.2% infusion at a rate of 3 mg/min using an infusion pump.
What is the rate in mL/hour?

Conversion of mL/hour back to a dose

48 You have dopexamine 50 mg in 50 mL and the rate at which the pump is running equals 21 mL/hour. What dose is the pump delivering?
(Patient's weight = 88 kg)

Calculating the length of time for IV infusions

49 A 500 mL infusion of sodium chloride 0.9% is being given at a rate of 21 drops/min (Standard giving set).
How long will the infusion run at the specified rate?

50 A 250 mL infusion of sodium chloride 0.9% is being given at a rate of 42 mL/hr.
How long will the infusion run at the specified rate?

ANSWERS TO PROBLEMS

Basics

Long multiplication
1 315,270
2 394.24

Long division
3 112.25
4 30

Fractions
5 $\dfrac{5}{21}$

6 $\dfrac{9}{16}$

7 $\dfrac{4}{3}$

8 $\dfrac{20}{9}$

9 0.4
10 0.56 (0.5625)

Decimals
11 11.25
12 25

13 80

14 0.064

15 $\dfrac{6}{5}$

16 $\dfrac{3}{8}$

Roman numerals

17 7

18 9

Powers

19 30,000

20 5×10^6

Per cent and percentages

21 70 g

22 40%

Units and equivalences

Units of weight

23 62.5 micrograms

24 0.6 kilograms

25 0.05 micrograms

Units of volume

26 150 millilitres

Units of amount of substance

27 360 millimoles

Drug strengths or concentrations

Percentage concentration

28 4.5 g

mg/mL concentrations

29 50 mg/5 mL

'I in ...' concentrations or ratio strengths

30 1 mg

Parts per million (ppm) strengths

31 0.7 mg

Dosage calculations

Calculating the number of tablets or capsules required

32 Three furosemide 40 mg tablets

Drug dosage
33 32 mg
34 219 mcg/min
35 2.325 mg

Calculating dosages
36 14 mL
37 3 mL
38 7.5 mL
39 4 ampoules

Paediatric calculations
40 9 mL
41 4.6 mL

Prescribing
42 Two 500 mL bottles (840 mL)
43 £3.36 (3 × £1.12)

Infusion rate calculations

Calculation of drip rates
44 27.7 drops/min (rounded to 28 drops/min)
45 15.625 drops/min (rounded to 16 drops/min)

Conversion of dosages to mL/hour
46 4.5 mL/hour
47 90 mL/hour

Conversion of mL/hour back to a dose
48 3.98 mcg/kg/min (approx 4 mcg/kg/min)

Calculating the length of time for IV infusions
49 7.94 hours (approx 8 hours)
50 5.95 hours (approx 6 hours)

PART I: Mathematics

1 BASICS

OBJECTIVES

At the end of this chapter, you should be familiar with the following:

- Arithmetic symbols
- Basic maths
  - Long multiplication
  - Long division
  - Mathematical tips and tricks
- Rules of arithmetic
- Fractions and decimals
  - Reducing or simplifying fractions
  - Equivalent fractions
  - Adding and subtracting fractions
  - Multiplying fractions
  - Dividing fractions
  - Converting fractions to decimals
  - Multiplying decimals
  - Dividing decimals
  - Rounding of decimal numbers
  - Converting decimals to fractions
- Roman numerals
- Powers or exponentials

KEY POINTS

Basic arithmetic rules

- Simple basic rules exist when adding (+), subtracting (−), multiplying (×), and dividing (/ or ÷) numbers – these are known as operations.
- The acronym BODMAS can be used to remember the correct order of operations:

B	Do calculations in **brackets** first. When you have more than one set of brackets, do the inner brackets first.
O	Next, do any **orders** (or powers).
D and **M**	Do the **division** and **multiplication** in order from left to right.
A and **S**	Do the **addition** and **subtraction** in order from left to right.

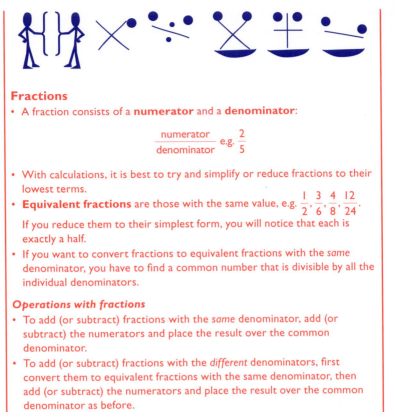

Fractions

- A fraction consists of a **numerator** and a **denominator**:

$$\frac{\text{numerator}}{\text{denominator}} \text{ e.g. } \frac{2}{5}$$

- With calculations, it is best to try and simplify or reduce fractions to their lowest terms.
- **Equivalent fractions** are those with the same value, e.g. $\frac{1}{2}, \frac{3}{6}, \frac{4}{8}, \frac{12}{24}$.

  If you reduce them to their simplest form, you will notice that each is exactly a half.
- If you want to convert fractions to equivalent fractions with the *same* denominator, you have to find a common number that is divisible by all the individual denominators.

Operations with fractions

- To add (or subtract) fractions with the *same* denominator, add (or subtract) the numerators and place the result over the common denominator.
- To add (or subtract) fractions with the *different* denominators, first convert them to equivalent fractions with the same denominator, then add (or subtract) the numerators and place the result over the common denominator as before.
- To multiply fractions, multiply the numerators and the denominators.
- To divide fractions, invert the second fraction and multiply (as above).
- To convert a fraction to a decimal, divide the numerator by the denominator.

Decimals

- When multiplying or dividing decimals, ensure that the decimal point is placed in the correct place.
- Rounding up or down of decimals:
    If the number after the decimal point is *4 or less*, then ignore it, i.e. **round down**.
    If the number after the decimal point is *5 or more*, then *add 1* to the whole number, i.e. **round up**.

Roman numerals

- In Roman numerals letters are used to designate numbers.

Powers or exponentials

- Powers or exponentials are a convenient way of writing large or small numbers:

  A positive power or exponent (e.g. 10^5) means *multiply* by the number of times of the power or exponent.

  A negative power or exponent (e.g. 10^{-5}) means *divide* by the number of times of the power or exponent.

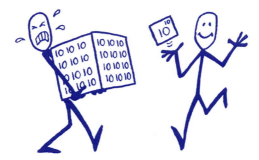

Using a calculator

- Ensure that numbers are entered correctly when using a calculator; if necessary, read the manual.

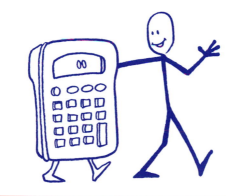

INTRODUCTION

Before dealing with any drug calculations, we will briefly go over a few basic mathematical concepts that may be helpful in some calculations.

This chapter is designed for those who might want to refresh their memories, particularly those who are returning to healthcare after a long absence.

You can skip some parts, or all, of this chapter. Alternatively, you can refer back to any part of this chapter as you are working through the rest of the book.

ARITHMETIC SYMBOLS

The following is a table of mathematical symbols generally used in textbooks. The list is not exhaustive, but covers common symbols you may come across.

SYMBOL	MEANING
+	plus or positive; add in calculations
−	minus or negative; subtract in calculations
±	plus or minus; positive or negative
×	multiply by
/ or ÷	divide by
=	equal to
≠	not equal to
≡	identically equal to
≈	approximately equal to
>	greater than
<	less than
≯	not greater than
≮	not less than
≤	equal to or less than
≥	equal to or greater than
%	per cent
Σ	sum of

BASIC MATHS

As a refresher, we will look at basic maths. This is quite useful if you don't have a calculator handy and can also help you understand how to perform drug calculations from first principles.

First, we will look at long multiplication and division.

Long multiplication

There are various methods for multiplying numbers – many based on ancient techniques. A quick Internet search will find many of these – ancient Egyptian; Russian peasant; Napier's grids/rods or Gelosia method, and using grids or boxes. Below is the traditional method for multiplication which many of you will remember from school. It relies on splitting numbers into their individual parts (hundreds, tens and units, etc).

Traditional method

To calculate 456 × 78:

```
H   T   U    First line up the numbers into hundreds (H), tens (T),
4   5   6    and units (U).
×   7   8
_____
_____
```

When using the traditional method, you multiply the number on the top row by the units and the tens separately, and then add the two together. In this case: 8 units and 7 tens.

First, multiply the numbers in the top row by the units (8), i.e. 8 × 6. Eight times 6 equals 48. Write the 8 in the units column and carry over the 4 to the tens column:

```
H   T   U
4   5   6
×   7   8
_____
        8
    4
```

Next, multiply by the next number in the top row, i.e. 8 × 5, which equals 40. Also add on the 4 that was carried over from the last step – this makes a total of 44. Write the 4 in the tens column and carry over the 4 to the hundreds column:

```
H   T   U
4   5   6
×   7   8
_____
    4   8
4   4
```

Next, multiply by the next number in the top row, i.e. 8 × 4, which equals 32. Also add on the 4 that was carried over from the last step – this makes a total of 36. Write down 36. You don't need to carry the 3, as there are no more numbers to multiply on this line:

```
Th  H   T   U
    4   5   6
×   7   8
_____
3   6   4   8
    4   4
```

Now we have to multiply by the tens. First, add a zero on the right-hand side of the next row. This is because we want to multiply by 70 (7 tens), which is the same as multiplying by 10 and by 7:

Th	H	T	U
	4	5	6
	×	7	8
3	6	4	8
			0

Multiply as before – this time it is 7 × 6, which equals 42. Place the 2 next to the zero and carry over the 4 to the hundreds column:

Th	H	T	U
	4	5	6
	×	7	8
3	6	4	8
		2	0
	4		

Next, multiply 7 × 5, which equals 35, and add on the 4 carried over to make a total of 39. Write down the 9 and carry over the 3:

Th	H	T	U
	4	5	6
	×	7	8
3	6	4	8
	9	2	0
3	4		

Finally, multiply 7 × 4, which equals 28. Add the 3 to equal 31 and write down 31. You don't need to carry the 3, as there are no more numbers to multiply on this line:

Th	H	T	U
	4	5	6
	×	7	8
	3	6	4	8
3	**1**	9	2	0

Begin adding up. Now you're done with multiplying; you just need to add together 3,648 and 31,920. Write a plus sign to remind you of this:

```
        Th  H  T  U
            4  5  6
          ×    7  8
        ─────────────
         3  6  4  8
   +  3  1  9  2  0
        ─────────────
      3  5  5  6  8
        ─────────────
           1
```

As before, carry over numbers (if necessary) when adding together.

You should get a final answer of 35,568.

For numbers of more than two digits, follow these steps: first multiply the top number by the units, then add a zero and multiply by the tens, then add two zeros and multiply by the hundreds, then add three zeros and multiply by the thousands, and so on. Add up all the numbers at the end.

Decimal numbers can be multiplied using this method. When dealing with decimal numbers, you have to ensure that the decimal point is placed correctly. Otherwise the steps you follow are the same as before (see *Decimals* later).

Long division

As with multiplication, dividing large numbers can be daunting. But if the process is broken down into several steps, it is made a lot easier.

Before we start, a brief mention of the terms sometimes used might be helpful. These are:

$$\frac{\text{dividend}}{\text{divisor}} = \text{quotient (answer)}$$

or

$$\text{divisor} \, \overline{)\text{dividend}}^{\text{quotient \quad (answer)}}$$

The process is as follows.

WORKED EXAMPLE

Divide 3,612 by 14:

$$14\overline{)3\ 6\ 1\ 2}$$

Long division works from left to right. First, look at 14 – it is a 2-digit number, it will not go into the first figure (i.e. the one on the left, which is 3). Obviously dividing 14 into 3 goes zero times or will not go. So we then consider the next number (6) with the 3 to give us 36 – this is greater than 14 (if it wasn't, we would have added successive numbers until a number greater than 14 is found). We then ask the question how many times can 14 go into 36? Twice 14 would equal 28; three times 14 would equal 42. So, the answer is 2.

14 into 36 goes 2.
Multiply 2 × 14.
Subtract the 28 from 36.

$$14 \overline{)3\ 6\ 1\ 2} \\ \quad\quad 2\ 8 \\ \quad\quad\ 8$$

Bring down the next digit (1).

$$14 \overline{)3\ 6\ 1\ 2} \\ \quad\quad 2\ 8\downarrow \\ \quad\quad\ 8\ 1$$

Then start the process again.

Divide 14 into 81. Once again, there is no exact number, 5 is the nearest number (6 would be too much). (If you are having trouble a quicker method would be to write down the 14 times table before starting the division.)

14 × 1 = 14
14 × 2 = 28
14 × 3 = 42
14 × 4 = 56
14 × 5 = 70
14 × 6 = 84
14 × 7 = 98
14 × 8 = 112
14 × 9 = 126
14 × 10 = 140

14 into 81 goes 5.
Multiply 14 × 5.
Subtract the 70 from 81.

$$14 \overline{)3\ 6\ 1\ 2} \\ \quad\quad 2\ 8 \\ \quad\quad\ 8\ 1 \\ \quad\quad\ 7\ 0 \\ \quad\quad\ 1\ 1$$

Bring down the next digit (2).

$$14 \overline{)3\ 6\ 1\ 2} \\ \quad\quad 2\ 8 \\ \quad\quad\ 8\ 1 \\ \quad\quad\ 7\ 0\downarrow \\ \quad\quad\ 1\ 1\ 2$$

$14 \times 1 = 14$		
$14 \times 2 = 28$		$14\overline{)3\ 6\ 1\ 2}$ $\ \ 2\ 5\ 8$
$14 \times 3 = 42$		
$14 \times 4 = 56$		
$14 \times 5 = 70$		
$14 \times 6 = 84$	14 into 112 goes 8.	
$14 \times 7 = 98$	Multiply 14×8.	
$14 \times 8 = 112$	Subtract $112 - 112$.	
$14 \times 9 = 126$		
$14 \times 10 = 140$	Answer = 258	

$$14\overline{)\begin{array}{r} 2\ 5\ 8 \\ \hline 3\ 6\ 1\ 2 \\ 2\ 8 \\ \hline 8\ 1 \\ 7\ 0 \\ \hline 1\ 1\ 2 \\ 1\ 1\ 2 \\ \hline 0 \end{array}}$$

If there was a remainder at the end of the units then you would bring down a zero as the next number and place a decimal point in the answer.

WORKED EXAMPLE

23 divided by 17:

$$17\overline{)2\ 3}$$

Firstly, divide the 17 into the first figure (i.e. the one on the left, which is 2). Obviously dividing 17 into 2 goes zero times or will not go. So we then consider the next number (3) and ask the question how many times can 17 go into 23? Obviously the answer is once; twice 17 would equal 34. So, the answer is 1.

17 into 23 goes 1.
Multiply 1×17.
Subtract the 17 from 23.
So the answer is 1 remainder 6.

$$17\overline{)\begin{array}{r} 1 \\ \hline 2\ 3 \\ 1\ 7 \\ \hline 6 \end{array}}$$

This could also be expressed as $1\dfrac{6}{17}$, but we would calculate to 2 or more decimal places.

We can consider 23 being the same as 23.00000; therefore, we can continue to divide the number:

$$17\overline{)\begin{array}{r} 1\ . \\ \hline 2\ 3\ .\ 0 \\ 1\ 7\ \ \downarrow \\ \hline 6\ \ 0 \end{array}}$$

Bring down the zero and put decimal point in the answer.

Then start the process again:

| 17 × 1 = 17 |
| 17 × 2 = 34 |
| 17 × 3 = 51 |
| 17 × 4 = 68 | 17 into 60 goes 3.
| 17 × 5 = 85 | Multiply 3 × 17.
| 17 × 6 = 102 | Subtract the 51 from 60.

```
              1 . 3
     17)2 3 . 0  0
        1 7
          6   0
          5   1
              9
```

Bring down the next zero.

And again repeat the process until there is no remainder or enough decimal places have been reached:

| 17 × 1 = 17 |
| 17 × 2 = 34 |
| 17 × 3 = 51 |
| 17 × 4 = 68 |
| 17 × 5 = 85 |
| 17 × 6 = 102 |

```
              1 . 3 5 2
     17)2 3 . 0 0 0
        1 7
          6   0
          5   1
              9 0
              8 5
                5 0
                3 4
                1 6
```

17 into 50 goes 2.
Multiply 2 × 17.
Subtract the 34 from 50.

If we were working to 2 decimal points, then our answer would be 1.35 (see rounding of decimals later in the chapter).

Mathematical tricks and tips

An in-depth study of mathematics would reveal that certain patterns occur which can be used to our advantage to make calculations a lot easier. Below are a few examples which may be helpful (an Internet search for 'mathematical tricks and tips' will give you many more examples).

Multiplication tips

The following is just manipulation of numbers by splitting the multiplication into smaller easier steps; you could probably devise your own.

Multiplying by 5

Multiply by 10 and divide by 2.

Multiplying by 6
Split into two steps – multiply by 3 and then by 2.

Multiplying by 9
Multiply by 10 and subtract the original number.

Multiplying by 12
Multiply by 10 and add twice the original number.

Multiplying by 13
Multiply by 3 and add 10 times original number.

Multiplying by 14
Split into two steps – multiply by 7 and then by 2.

Multiplying by 15
Multiply by 10 and add 5 times the original number.

Multiplying by 16
You can double four times, or split into two steps – multiply by 8 and then by 2.

Multiplying by 17
Multiply by 7 and add 10 times original number.

Multiplying by 18
Multiply by 2, add a zero at the end of the answer, and finally subtract twice the original number (which is obvious from the first step).

Multiplying by 19
Multiply by 2, add a zero at the end of the answer, and finally subtract the original number.

Multiplying by 24
Split into two steps – multiply by 8 and then by 3.

Multiplying by 27
Multiply by 3, add a zero at the end of the answer, and finally subtract 3 times the original number (which is obvious from the first step).

Multiplying by 45
Multiply by 5, add a zero at the end of the answer, and finally subtract 5 times the original number (which is obvious from the first step).

Multiplying by 90
Multiply by 9 (as above) and put a zero on the end.

Multiplying by 98
Multiply by 100 and subtract twice the original number.

Multiplying by 99
Multiply by 100 and subtract the original number.

Dividing tips
Try to simplify your sum to give smaller, more manageable numbers. For example:

$$525 \div 45$$

Both numbers are divisible by 5, so we can simplify by dividing by 5 to give

$$105 \div 9$$

Note both numbers are now divisible by 3, so we can simplify further by dividing each number by 3 to give:

$$35 \div 3$$

How can you spot that numbers can be simplified? The following are simple rules to see which numbers can be used to simplify any division sum.

Dividing by 2
All even numbers are divisible by 2.

Dividing by 3
Add up the digits to get a single number; if it is divisible by 3, then the number will be too.

Dividing by 4
If the last 2 digits of the number are divisible by 4, then the whole number is divisible by 4. However, it is probably easier to divide by 2 in several steps.

Dividing by 5
Numbers ending in a 5 or a 0 are always divisible by 5.

Dividing by 6

If the number is divisible by 3 and 2, then it is divisible by 6 as well.

Dividing by 7

Take the last digit, double it, then subtract the answer from the remaining numbers; if that number is divisible by 7, then the original number is too. For example:

> 203   Take the last number (3) and double it to give 6; subtract from the remaining numbers (20 − 6) to give 14. This number (14) is divisible by 7 and so must be the original number (203).

Dividing by 8

Remove the last digit and put to one side; double the remaining digits and then add the number you put aside – if the answer is divisible by 8, then the original is as well. However, it is probably easier to divide by 2 in several steps. For example:

> 208   Take the last number (8) and put to one side; double the remaining digits (20) to give 40, then add the original digit you put to one side (8): 40 + 8 = 48. This number is divisible by 8 and so must be the original number.

Dividing by 9

Add up all the digits until you get a single number; if it is 9, then the original number is divisible by 9.

Note: It will also be divisible by 3.

Dividing by 10

Numbers ending in a 0 are always divisible by 10 (simply remove the zero at the end).

RULES OF ARITHMETIC

Now that we have covered basic multiplication and division, in what order should we perform an arithmetic sum?

Consider the sum: 3 + 4 × 6

- Do we add 3 and 4 together, and then multiply by 6, to give 42? or
- Do we multiply 4 by 6, and then add 3, to give 27?

There are two possible answers depending upon how you would solve the above sum – which one is right?

The correct answer is 27.

Why is this? Rules were developed to ensure that everyone follows the same way to solve problems – known as rules for the order of operations.

Rules for the order of operations

The processes of adding (+), subtracting (−), multiplying (×) and dividing (/or ÷) numbers are known as **operations**. When you have complicated sums to do, you have to follow simple rules known as the **order of operations**. Initially people agreed on an order in which mathematical operations should be performed, and this has been universally adopted.

The acronym **BODMAS** is used to remember the correct order of operations. Each letter stands for a common mathematical operation; the **order** of the letter matches the **order** in which we do the mathematical operations. You can even make up your own phrase if you wish, to remember the correct order of operations.

B	stands for	**Brackets**	e.g. (3 + 4)
O	stands for	**pOwers**	e.g. 2^3
D	stands for	**Division**	e.g. 6 ÷ 3
M	stands for	**Multiplication**	e.g. 3 × 4
A	stands for	**Addition**	e.g. 3 + 4
S	stands for	**Subtraction**	e.g. 4 − 3

TIP BOX

The basic rule is to work from **left** to **right**.

For the types of calculations that you will encounter every day you need to remember that division/multiplication are done before addition/subtraction.

Consider the following simple sum: 10 − 3 + 2.

Remember – work from left to right.

The first operation we come across is subtraction, so this is done first:

$$10 - 3 = 7$$

Then addition:

$$7 + 2 = 9$$

So 9 is the right answer.

Now consider this sum: 3 + 5 × 4

Remember – work from left to right.

The first operation we come across is addition, but we notice that the next one is multiplication. Remembering the order of operations – multiplication is done before addition. So, multiplication is done before addition:

$$5 \times 4 = 20$$

Then addition:

$$3 + 20 = 23$$

So 23 is the right answer.

B	Calculations in brackets are done first. When you have more than one set of brackets, do the inner brackets first.
O	Next, any powers (or exponentiation) must be done. You are unlikely to deal with powers in day-to-day calculations, but calculators use this to display large numbers.
D and **M**	Do the multiplication and division in order from left to right.
A and **S**	Do the addition and subtraction in order from left to right.

WORKED EXAMPLE

If we look at the example from Appendix 5 (calculating creatinine clearance), we can see that it is quite a complicated sum:

$$CrCl \text{ (mL/min)} = \frac{1.23 \times (140 - 67) \times 72}{125} = 51.7$$

In the top line, the sum within the brackets is done first, i.e. $(140 - 67)$, then we multiply by 1.23 and then by 72.

Thus, $(140 - 67) = 73$, so the sum is $1.23 \times 73 \times 72 = 6,464.88$.

Then divide by 125 to give the answer of 51.7 to one decimal place.

TIP BOX

If there is a 'line', work out the top, then the bottom, and finally divide.

FRACTIONS AND DECIMALS

A basic knowledge of fractions and decimals is helpful since they are involved in most calculations. It is important to know how to multiply and divide fractions and decimals as well as to be able to convert from a fraction to a decimal and vice versa. An understanding of fractions will also demonstrate numeracy skills.

Fractions

Before we look at fractions, a few points are defined to make explanations easier.

Definition of a fraction

A fraction is part of a whole number or one number divided by another.

For example: $\frac{2}{5}$ is a fraction and means 2 parts of 5 (where 5 is the whole).

The number above the line is called the **numerator**; the word is derived from the Latin verb to count (*enumero*). It 'counts' or indicates the number of parts of the whole number that are being used (i.e. 2 in the above example).

The number below the line is called the **denominator**; the word is derived from the Latin word for name (*nomen*). It 'names' or indicates the value of the fraction, and it indicates the number of parts into which the whole is divided. (i.e. 5 in the above example).

Thus in the above example, the whole has been divided into 5 equal parts and you are dealing with 2 parts of the whole.

$$\frac{2 \quad \text{numerator}}{5 \quad \text{denominator}}$$

It can also be written as 2/5.

If the denominator (bottom number) is *less* or *smaller than* the numerator (top number) then the fraction is *greater* than 1.

If the denominator (bottom number) is *more* or *bigger than* the numerator (top number) then the fraction is *less* than 1.

Simplifying (reducing) fractions

When you haven't a calculator handy, it is often easier to work with fractions that have been simplified, or reduced to their lowest terms. We have encountered this earlier when dealing with long division. To reduce a fraction, choose any number that divides exactly into the numerator (number on the top) and the denominator (number on the bottom).

A fraction is said to have been reduced to its lowest terms when it is no longer possible to divide the numerator and denominator by the same number. This process of converting or reducing a fraction to its simplest form is called **cancellation**.

Remember – reducing or simplifying a fraction to its lowest terms does not change the value of the fraction.

Calculations with fractions (addition, subtraction, multiplication, or division) are made easier if the fraction is simplified first.

WORKED EXAMPLE

1. $\dfrac{\dfrac{\cancel{15}}{\cancel{25}}}{5} = \dfrac{3}{5}$

3

2. 3

$\dfrac{\dfrac{\cancel{27}}{\cancel{135}}}{\dfrac{\cancel{315}}{\cancel{63}}} = \dfrac{3}{7}$

7

The 15 and 25 are divided by 5.

a) The 135 and 315 are divided by 5.
b) The 27 and 63 are divided by 9.

Remember:

- Any number that ends in 0 or 5 is divisible by 5.
- Any even number is divisible by 2.
- There can be more than one step (see the example on the right).

If you have a calculator, then there is no need to reduce fractions to their lowest terms: the calculator does all the hard work for you.

Equivalent fractions

Consider the following fractions:

$$\frac{1}{2} \quad \frac{3}{6} \quad \frac{4}{8} \quad \frac{12}{24}$$

Each of the above fractions has the same value: they are called **equivalent** fractions.

If you reduce them to their simplest form, you will notice that each is exactly a half.

Now consider the following fractions:

If you want to convert them to equivalent fractions with the **same** denominator, you have to find a common number that is divisible by all the individual denominators. For example, in the above case, multiply each denominator by 2, 3, 4, etc. until the smallest common number is found, as illustrated in this table:

	3	4	6
× 2	6	8	12
× 3	9	12	18
× 4	12	16	24

In this case, the common denominator is 12. For each fraction, multiply the numbers above and below the line by the common multiple. So for the first fraction, multiply the numbers above and below the line by 4; for the second multiply them by 3; and for the third multiply them by 2. So the fractions become:

$$\frac{1}{3} \times \frac{4}{4} = \frac{4}{12} \text{ and } \frac{1}{4} \times \frac{3}{3} = \frac{3}{12} \text{ and } \frac{1}{6} \times \frac{2}{2} = \frac{2}{12}$$

$$\frac{1}{3}, \frac{1}{4} \text{ and } \frac{1}{6} \text{ equal } \frac{4}{12}, \frac{3}{12} \text{ and } \frac{2}{12}, \text{ respectively.}$$

Adding and subtracting fractions

To add (or subtract) fractions with the *same* denominator, add (or subtract) the numerators and place the result over the common denominator, i.e.

$$\frac{14}{32} + \frac{7}{32} - \frac{4}{32} = \frac{14 + 7 - 4}{32} = \frac{17}{32}$$

To add (or subtract) fractions with *different* denominators, first convert them to equivalent fractions with the same denominator, then add (or subtract) the numerators and place the result over the common denominator as before, i.e.

$$\frac{1}{4} - \frac{1}{6} + \frac{1}{3} = \frac{3}{12} - \frac{2}{12} + \frac{4}{12} = \frac{3 - 2 + 4}{12} = \frac{5}{12}$$

Sometimes, when converting to equivalent fractions, the resultant fractions may have large numbers. To make them easier to deal with, see if you can simplify the fraction in any way.

Multiplying fractions

It is quite easy to multiply fractions. You simply multiply all the numbers above the line (the numerators) and the numbers below the line (the denominators).

For example:

$$\frac{2}{5} \times \frac{3}{7} = \frac{2 \times 3}{5 \times 7} = \frac{6}{35}$$

However, it may be possible to simplify the fraction before multiplying, i.e.

$$\frac{\overset{3}{\cancel{9}}}{\underset{5}{\cancel{15}}} \times \frac{2}{5} = \frac{3 \times 2}{5 \times 5} = \frac{6}{25}$$

In this case, the first fraction has been reduced to its lowest terms by dividing both the numerator and denominator by 3.

You can also reduce both fractions by dividing diagonally by a common number, i.e.

$$\frac{\overset{2}{\cancel{6}}}{7} \times \frac{5}{\underset{3}{\cancel{9}}} = \frac{2 \times 5}{7 \times 3} = \frac{10}{21}$$

In this case, in both fractions there is a number that is divisible by 3 (6 and 9).

Dividing fractions
Sometimes it may be necessary to divide fractions. You will probably encounter fractions expressed or written like this:

$$\frac{\frac{2}{5}}{\frac{3}{7}} \text{ which is the same as } \frac{2}{5} \div \frac{3}{7}$$

In this case, you simply invert the second fraction (or the bottom one) and multiply, i.e.

$$\frac{2}{5} \times \frac{7}{3} = \frac{2 \times 7}{5 \times 3} = \frac{14}{15}$$

If, after inverting, you see that reduction or cancellation is possible, you can do this before multiplying. For example:

$$\frac{5}{2} \div \frac{25}{8}$$

This becomes:

$$\frac{\overset{1}{\cancel{5}}}{\underset{1}{\cancel{2}}} \times \frac{\overset{4}{\cancel{8}}}{\underset{5}{\cancel{25}}} = \frac{1 \times 4}{1 \times 5} = \frac{4}{5}$$

> **TIP BOX**
>
> When doing any sum involving fractions, simplifying the fractions will make the calculation easier.

Converting fractions to decimals
This is quite easy to do. You simply divide the top number (numerator) by the bottom number (denominator).
   If we use our original example:

$$\frac{2}{5} \text{ which can be rewritten as } 2 \div 5 \text{ or } 5\overline{)2}$$

$$
\begin{array}{r}
0.4 \\
5\,\overline{)2.0} \\
\underline{2.0} \\
0
\end{array}
$$

It is important to place the decimal point in the correct position, usually after the number being divided (in this case it is 2).

Decimals

Decimals in the form of digital displays may be encountered on a regular basis – for example with infusion and syringe pumps. Understanding decimals is therefore an important part of numeracy skills.

Pierce *et al.* (2008) noted that some nurses had difficulty interpreting decimal numbers because their understanding of decimals was inadequate – for example, thinking that 4.63 is bigger than 4.8 (because 63 is bigger than 8).

Problems with decimals can lead to medication errors. Lesar (2002) looked at medication errors over an 18-month period; 200 were tenfold medication errors (61% were overdoses) due to a misplaced decimal point in 43.5% of cases.

Similarly, another study (Doherty and McDonnell 2012) looked at tenfold medication errors – this time over a 5-year period in a paediatric hospital. Errors of dose calculation due to omitted or misplaced decimal points and confusion with zeros were frequent contributing factors.

Decimals describe tenths of a number, i.e. in terms of 10. A decimal number consists of a decimal point and numbers to both the left and right of that decimal point. Just as whole numbers have positions for units, tens, hundreds, etc. so do decimal numbers, but on *both* sides of the decimal point, i.e.

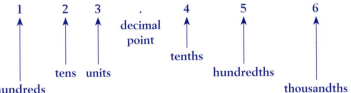

Numbers to the **left** of the **decimal point** are **greater than one**.
Numbers to the **right** of the **decimal point** are **less than one**.

Thus:

0.25 is a fraction of 1

1.25 is 1 plus a fraction of 1

Multiplying decimals

Decimals are multiplied in the same way as whole numbers except there is a decimal point to worry about. If you are not using a calculator, remember to put the decimal point in the correct place in the answer.

Consider the sum: 0.65×0.75.

At first, it looks a bit daunting with the decimal points, but the principles covered earlier with long multiplication also apply here. You just have to be careful with the decimal point.

$$
\begin{array}{r}
0.6\,5 \\
\times\ 0.7\,5 \\
\hline
\end{array}
$$

In essence, you are multiplying '65' by '75':

$$
\begin{array}{r}
0.\mathbf{6\,5} \\
\times\ 0.\mathbf{7\,5} \\
\hline
\end{array}
$$

As before, multiply the top row first by the number after the decimal point (part of a unit), then by the units, tens, etc. as appropriate.

First, multiply the top row by 5:

$$
\begin{array}{r}
0.6\,5 \\
\times\ 0.7\,5 \\
\hline
5 \\
\hline
2 \\
\end{array}
$$

Five times five equals 25, write the five under the Units column and carry over the 2 to the Tens column

Continue as before until you have multiplied all the numbers in the top row:

$$
\begin{array}{r}
0.6\,5 \\
\times\ 0.7\,5 \\
\hline
3\ \ 2\,5 \\
\hline
2 \\
\end{array}
$$

Next, multiply the top row by 7 (don't forget to place a zero at the end of the second line):

$$
\begin{array}{r}
0.6\,5 \\
\times\ 0.7\,5 \\
\hline
3\ \ 2\,5 \\
4\,5\ \ 5\,0 \\
\hline
3 \\
\end{array}
$$

Now add the two lines together:

$$
\begin{array}{r}
0\,.\,6\;5 \\
\times\,0\,.\,7\;5 \\
\hline
3\;\;\;2\;5 \\
4\;5\;\;5\;0 \\
\hline
4\;8\;\;7\;5
\end{array}
$$

Finally, we have to decide where to place the decimal point. The decimal point is placed as many places to the **left** as there are numbers after it in the sum (i.e. in this case there are four):

$$
0\,.\,6\;5 \times 0\,.\,7\;5
$$
$$
I\;2\qquad 3\;4 = 4
$$

Therefore in the answer, the decimal point is moved four places to the *left*.

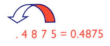

$$.\,4\,8\,7\,5 = 0.4875$$

Multiplying by multiples of 10

To multiply a decimal by multiples of 10 (100, 1,000, etc.) you simply move the decimal point the number of places to the *right* as there are zeros in the number you are multiplying by.
For example:

NUMBER TO MULTIPY BY	NUMBER OF ZEROS	MOVE THE DECIMAL POINT TO THE RIGHT
10	1	1 place
100	2	2 places
1,000	3	3 places
10,000	4	4 places

For example:

$$54.6 \times 1,000$$

Move the decimal point THREE places to the RIGHT. (There are THREE zeros in the number it is being multiplied by.)

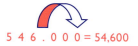

5 4 6 . 0 0 0 = 54,600

References

Pierce RU, Steinle VA, Stacey C, Widjaja W. Understanding decimal numbers: a foundation for correct calculations. *International Journal of Nursing Education Scholarship* 2008 (Jan); 5(1): 1–15.

Lesar T. Tenfold medication dose prescribing errors. *Annals of Pharmacotherapy* 2002 (Dec); 36(12): 1833–1839.

Doherty C, McDonnell C. Tenfold medication errors: 5 years' experience at a university-affiliated pediatric hospital. *Pediatrics* 2012 (May); 129(5): 915–924.

Dividing decimals

Once again, decimals are divided in the same way as whole numbers except there is a decimal point to worry about.

A recap of the terms sometimes used is given here.

$$\frac{\text{dividend}}{\text{divisor}} = \text{quotient (answer)}$$

or

$$\text{divisor} \overline{)\text{dividend}}^{\text{quotient} \quad \text{(answer)}}$$

WORKED EXAMPLE

Consider $\frac{34.8}{4}$ which can be rewritten as $34.8 \div 4$ or $4\overline{)3\ 4\ .\ 8}$

The decimal point in the answer (quotient) is placed directly above the decimal point in the dividend:

$$4\overline{)3\ 4\ .\ 8}^{\quad\ \ .}$$

First, divide the 4 into the first figure (the one on the left, which is 3). Obviously dividing 4 into 3 goes zero times or will not go. So we then consider the next number (4) and ask: How many times can 4 go into 34? Eight times 4 equals 32; nine times 4 equals 36. So, the answer is 8.

Divide 4 into 34; it goes 8 times.

$$\begin{array}{r} 8 \\ 4\overline{)3\ 4\ .\ 8} \\ 3\ 2 \\ \hline 2\ \ 8 \end{array}$$

Multiply 4 × 8.
Subtract 32 from 34.
Bring down the next number (8).

Place the decimal point in the answer (quotient) above the point in the dividend.
　　Then start the process again:

$$\begin{array}{r} 8\ .\ 7 \\ 4\overline{)3\ 4\ .\ 8} \\ 3\ 2 \\ \hline 2\ \ 8 \\ 2\ \ 8 \\ \hline 0 \end{array}$$

4 into 28 goes 7 times.
Multiply 4 × 7.
Subtract 28 from 28.

What do we do when both the divisor and dividend are decimals?

WORKED EXAMPLE

Consider $\dfrac{1.55}{0.2}$ which can be rewritten as $1.55 \div 0.2$ or $0.2\overline{)1\ .\ 5\ 5}$

First make the **divisor** equal to a **whole number**; in this case, move the decimal point **one** place to the **right**. Then move the decimal point in the **dividend** the **same number** of places to the **right**.
In this case:

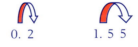

0. 2　　　　1. 5 5

Which is equal to

$$2\overline{)1\ 5\ .\ 5}$$

The decimal point in the answer (quotient) is placed directly above the decimal point in the dividend.

$$2\overline{)1\ 5\ .\ 5}$$

As before, perform the same steps as for example one:

2 into 15 goes 7 times.
Multiply 2 × 7.
Subtract 14 from 15.

```
        7
    2)1 5 . 5
      1 4
        1
```

Bring down the next number (5).

```
        7
    2)1 5 . 5
      1 4    ↓
        1  5
```

2 into 15 goes 7 times.
Multiply 2 × 7.
Subtract 14 from 15.

```
        7 . 7
    2)1 5 . 5
      1 4
        1  5
        1  4
           1
```

Place the decimal point in the answer (quotient) above the point in the dividend:

```
        7 . 7
    2)1 5 . 5 0
      1 4      |
        1  5   |
        1  4  ↓
           1 0
```

Bring down a zero (0).

Repeat as before:

```
        7 . 7 5
    2)1 5 . 5 0
      1 4
        1  5
        1  4
           1 0
```

2 into 10 goes 5 times.
Multiply 2 × 5.
Subtract 10 from 10.

```
           1 0
              0
```

So the answer is 7.75.

Dividing by multiples of 10

To divide a decimal by a multiple of 10, you simply move the decimal point the number of places to the **left** as there are number of zeros in the number you are dividing by.

NUMBER TO DIVIDE BY	NUMBER OF ZEROS	MOVE THE DECIMAL POINT TO THE LEFT
10	1	1 place
100	2	2 places
1,000	3	3 places
10,000	4	4 places

For example:

$\dfrac{54.6}{1,000}$ Move the decimal point *three* places to the *left*. (There are *three* zeros in the bottom number.)

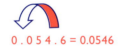

0 . 0 5 4 . 6 = 0.0546

Rounding of decimal numbers

Sometimes it is necessary to 'round up' or 'round down' a decimal number to a whole number. This is particularly true in drip rate calculations because it is impossible to give a part of a drop.

If the number after the decimal point is 4 or less, then ignore it, i.e. round down.

For example: 31.25: The number after the decimal point is 2 (which is less than 4), so it becomes 31.

If the number after the decimal point is 5 or more, then add 1 to the whole number, i.e. round up.

For example: 41.67: The number after the decimal point is 6 (which is more than 5), so it becomes 42.

Sometimes, you might have to 'round' decimals to two or more decimal places.

For example: 348. 648: We need to look at the third number after the decimal point (8); it is greater than 5, so the previous number (4) is 'rounded' up by 1 (i.e. 4 becomes 5).

It may be necessary to round to two decimal places when dealing with very small doses.

Converting decimals to fractions

It is unlikely that you would want to convert a decimal to a fraction in any calculation, but this is included here just in case.

- First you have to make the decimal a whole number by moving the decimal point to the RIGHT, i.e.

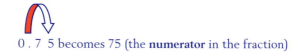

0 . 7 5 becomes 75 (the **numerator** in the fraction)

- Next divide by a multiple of 10 (the **denominator**) to make a fraction.

    The value of this multiple of 10 is determined by how many places to the **right** the decimal point has moved, i.e.

1 place = a *denominator* of 10

2 places = a *denominator* of 100

3 places = a *denominator* of 1,000

Thus in our example 0.75 becomes 75, i.e. the decimal point has moved 2 places to the *right*, so the denominator is 100:

$$\frac{75}{100}$$

The above can be simplified by dividing the numerator and denominator by 25:

$$= \frac{3}{4}$$

So the denominator will always either be 10, 100, 1,000 and so on.

$$0.3 = \frac{3}{10}$$

$$0.03 = \frac{3}{100}$$

$$0.003 = \frac{3}{1,000}$$

ROMAN NUMERALS

Although it is not recommended as best practice, Roman numerals are still commonly used when writing prescriptions. With Roman numerals, letters are used to designate numbers.

The following table explains the Roman numerals most commonly seen on prescriptions.

ROMAN NUMERAL	ORDINARY NUMBER
I (or i)	1
II (or ii)	2
III (or iii)	3
IV (or iv)	4
V (or v)	5
VI (or vi)	6
VII (or vii)	7
VIII (or viii)	8
IX (or ix)	9
X (or x)	10
L (or l)	50
C (or c)	100
D (or d)	500
M (or m)	1,000

Rules for reading Roman numerals

There are some simple rules for Roman numerals. It doesn't matter whether they are capital letters or small letters, the value is the same. The position of one letter relative to another is very important and determines the value of the numeral.

- **Rule 1:** Repeating a Roman numeral twice doubles its value; repeating it three times triples its value, e.g.

$$II = (I + I) = 2; III = (I + I + I) = 3$$

- **Rule 2:** The letters I can usually be repeated up to three times; the letter V is written once only, e.g.

$$III = 3 \text{ is correct}; IIII = 4 \text{ is not correct}$$

- **Rule 3:** When a smaller Roman numeral is placed after a larger one, add the two together, e.g.

$$VI = 5 + 1 = 6$$

- **Rule 4:** When a smaller Roman numeral is placed before a larger one, subtract the smaller numeral from the larger one, e.g.

$$IV = 5 - I = 4$$

- **Rule 5:** When a Roman numeral of a smaller value comes between two larger values, first apply the subtraction rule, and then add, e.g.

$$XIV = 10 + (5 - I) = 10 + 4 = 14$$

POWERS OR EXPONENTIALS

Powers or exponentials are a convenient way of writing very large or very small numbers. Powers of 10 are often used in scientific calculations.

Consider the following:

$$100,000 \text{ which is the same as } 10 \times 10 \times 10 \times 10 \times 10$$

Here you are multiplying by 10, five times. Instead of all these 10s, you can write:

$$10^5$$

We say this as '10 to the power of 5' or just '10 to the 5'. The small raised number 5 next to the 10 is known as the **power** or **exponent** – it tells you how many of the same number are being multiplied together.

$$10^5 \nwarrow \text{power or exponent}$$

We came across the terms power or exponent when looking at the rules of arithmetic earlier.

Now consider this:

$$0.000001 \text{ which is the same as } \frac{1}{10 \times 10 \times 10 \times 10 \times 10}$$

Here you are dividing by 10, five times. Instead of all these 10s, you can write:

$$10^{-5}$$

In this case, you will notice that there is a minus sign next to the power or exponent:

$$10^{-5} \nwarrow \text{minus power or exponent}$$

This is a **negative power** or **exponent** and is usually called '10 to the power of –5' or just '10 to the minus 5'.

In conclusion:

- A positive power or exponent means *multiply* by the number of times of the power or exponent.
- A negative power or exponent means *divide* by the number of times of the power or exponent.

You will probably come across powers used as in the following:

Lymphocytes as 3.5×10^9/L

This is known as the **standard index form**. It is useful when writing very big or very small numbers.

In standard form, a number is always written as: $A \times 10^n$.

'A' is always a number between 1 and 10, and 'n' tells us how many places to move the decimal point.

For example: 250,000,000 written in standard index form would be $2.5 \times 10,000,000$.

This can be rewritten as: $2.5 \times 10 \times 10 \times 10 \times 10 \times 10 \times 10 \times 10$ or 2.5×10^7.

This type of notation is the type seen on a scientific calculator when you are working with very large or very small numbers. It is a common and convenient way of describing numbers without having to write a lot of zeros.

Because you are dealing in 10s, you will notice that the 'number of zeros' you multiply or divide by is equal to the power.

You can convert from standard form to ordinary numbers, and back again. Have a look at these examples:

$$3 \times 10^5 = 3 \times 100,000 = 300,000$$
$$\left(\text{since } 10^5 = 10 \times 10 \times 10 \times 10 \times 10 = 100,000 - \text{i.e. 5 zeros} \right)$$

$$3,850,000 = 3.85 \times 1,000,000 = 3.85 \times 10^6 \text{ (i.e. 6 zeros)}$$

$$0.000567 = 5.67 \times 0.0001 = 5.67 \times 10^{-4}$$
$$\left(\text{since } 10^{-4} = \frac{1}{10} \times \frac{1}{10} \times \frac{1}{10} \times \frac{1}{10} = \frac{1}{10,000} - \text{i.e. 4 zeros} \right)$$

Make the first number between 1 and 10.

OBJECTIVES

At the end of this chapter, you should be familiar with the following:

- Sense of number and working from first principles
- Estimation of answers
- The 'one unit' rule
- Checking your answer – does it seem reasonable?
- Minimizing errors

SENSE OF NUMBER AND THE USE OF CALCULATORS OR FORMULAE

In all calculations, particularly those involving drugs, it is important to have some idea as to what the answer should be. You should be able to perform simple and straightforward calculations without the use of a calculator.

There is a risk that calculators and formulae will be used without a basic understanding of what the numbers being entered actually mean; consequently there is a potential for mistakes. Users may become deskilled in the basics of mathematics, and as a result, the ability to determine whether an answer is reasonable is lost, and potential errors are not noticed (McMullan 2010).

Working from first principles and using basic arithmetical skills allows you to have a 'sense of number' and reduces the risk of making mistakes.

The NMC *Standards for Medicines Management* (Feb 2008) states:

> The use of calculators to determine the volume or quantity of medication should not act as a substitute for arithmetical knowledge and skill.

To ensure that when pharmacists qualify they have basic arithmetical skills and this 'sense of number', the General Pharmaceutical Council does not allow the use of calculators in the registration exam. However, this does not mean that calculators should not be used – calculators can increase accuracy and can be helpful for complex calculations. But a calculator can only be as accurate as the information entered – calculators cannot indicate whether the numbers entered are correct or are in the correct order.

With any calculator, it is important to read the instructions and familiarize yourself with how it works. It is a good idea to first try some simple calculations you already know the answers to – this will allow you to get used to your calculator. Be sure that you check each entry on the display to make sure that you are entering the right numbers.

The belief that a calculator or a formula is infallible and that the answer it gives is automatically correct gives a false sense of security. It is important that you understand the process involved in any calculation so that you can judge whether the answer obtained is reasonable.

An article in the *Nursing Standard* in May 2008 also highlighted the fact that using formulae relies solely on arithmetic for an answer which is devoid of meaning and context. The article mentions that skill is required to extract the correct numbers from the clinical situation; place them correctly in the formula; perform the arithmetic; and translate the answer back to the clinical context to find the meaning of the number and thence the action to be taken (Wright 2008).

The advantage of working from first principles is that you can put your answer back into the correct clinical context.

You may have entered the numbers correctly into your formula or calculator and arrived at the correct answer of 1.2 – but what does it mean? You might mistakenly believe that you need to give 1.2 ampoules instead of 1.2 mL. Having a 'sense of number' helps to ensure that the answer is given in the correct clinical context.

References

McMullan M. Exploring the numeracy skills of nurses and students when performing drug calculations. *Nursing Times* 2010; 106(34): 10–12.

NMC. *Standards for Medicine Management* (2008). Nursing and Midwifery Council, London.

Wright K. Drug calculations part 1: a critique of the formula used by nurses. *Nursing Standard* 2008; 22(36): 40–42.

ESTIMATION OF ANSWERS

Looking at a drug calculation with a 'sense of number' means that we can often have a rough idea, or estimate, of the answer. It is important to be able to estimate the final answer in drug calculations, not only to ensure that the correct dose is given, but also to check that the prescribed dose is appropriate. Estimation skills are particularly helpful when calculations are somewhat complicated – estimating in steps helps to ensure that the final answer is correct.

Estimation is made easier with experience, but common sense should always be paramount. You are not trying to get the exact answer, but something that is an approximation.

The estimating process is basically simple – it is just manipulation of numbers to make calculations easier. Numbers can be:

- Rounded up or down – usually in multiples of fives or tens to give numbers that can be calculated easily. For example, 41 would be rounded down to 40, 23.5 to 20, and 148.75 rounded up to 150. Single-digit numbers can be left as they are (although 8 and 9 could be rounded up to 10).
- Halved or doubled in steps to make calculations easier.
- Reduced to a 'unit' dose, whether it's 1 mcg, 0.1 mcg, or 0.01 mcg, and used for multiples of dose.

There are no set rules for estimating, and several methods are available – pick the one most suited to you.

The following examples illustrate the principles involved. Don't forget – the answer is only an estimate. If you round *up* numbers, the estimated answer will be *more* than the actual answer. If you round *down* numbers, the estimated answer will be *less* than the actual answer.

1. You have 200 mg in 10 mL.
   From this, you can easily work out the following:
   100 mg – 5 mL (by halving)
   50 mg – 2.5 mL (by halving)
   150 mg – 7.5 mL (by addition; 100 mg + 50 mg and 5 mL + 2.5 mL)
2. You have 100 mg in 1 mL.
   From this, you can easily work out the following:
   500 mg – 5 mL (by multiplying by 5; 100 mg × 5 and 1 mL × 5)
   1 mg – 0.01 mL (unit dose by dividing by 100)
   200 mg – 2 mL (by doubling)

Throughout the book, in all the worked examples, we estimate answers using various techniques which will help you develop your own.

If estimation is not possible, then rely on experience and common sense. If your answer means that you would need 6 ampoules of an injection for your calculated dose, then common sense should dictate that this is not normal practice (see later: *Checking Your Answer – Does It Seem Reasonable?*).

THE 'ONE UNIT' RULE

Various methods are available for drug calculations – we will be using the 'one unit' rule throughout this book. Using it will allow you to work from first principles and have a 'sense of number'.

The rule works by proportion: What you do to one side of an equation, do the same to the other side. Because it works by proportion, the amounts remain equal. In whatever type of calculation you are doing, it is always best to make what you've got equal to *one* and then multiply by what you want – hence the name.

It is also important to assign units to the numbers at each step; in this way you will know exactly what the answer means and its clinical context.

The following example explains the concept more clearly. We use boxes in the form of a table to make the explanation easier.

If 12 apples cost £2.88 – how much would 5 apples cost?

If we have a 'sense of number' we can estimate our answer. Six apples would cost half of £2.88 which would be £1.44; 3 apples would cost half of that: 72p. So 5 apples would cost between 72p and £1.44; probably nearer the upper figure – say £1.30 as a guess.

Let's do the calculation using the 'one unit' rule.

Write down everything we know (don't forget to add the units for each number, in this case it will be 'apples' and '£'):

12 apples   cost   £2.88

Then write down what we want to know underneath:

12 apples   cost   £2.88
5 apples   cost   ?

We will write everything using boxes in the form of a table.

L		R
12 apples	cost	£2.88
5 apples	cost	?

The left side (column L) = what you know and what you want to know
   The right side (column R) = the known and unknown.

First calculate how much one of whatever you have (one unit) is equal to. This is done by proportion.

Make everything you know (column L) equal to 1 by dividing by 12:

$$\frac{12}{12} \text{ apples} = 1 \text{ apple}$$

As we have done this to one side of the equation (column L), we must do the same to the other side (column R):

$$\frac{£2.88}{12}$$

L		R
12 apples	cost	£2.88
$\dfrac{12}{12}$ apples = 1 apple	cost	$\dfrac{£2.88}{12}$

Next, multiply by what you want to know, in this case it is the cost of 5 apples.

So multiply 1 apple (column L) by 5 – don't forget, we have to do the same to the other side of the equation (column R).

L		R
12 apples	cost	£2.88
$\dfrac{12}{12}$ apples = 1 apple	cost	$\dfrac{£2.88}{12}$
5 apples = 1 × 5 = 5	cost	$\dfrac{£2.88}{12} \times 5 = £1.20$

So 5 apples would cost £1.20.

Working from first principles ensures that the correct units are used and that there is no confusion as to what the answer actually means.

Checking with our original estimation: 5 apples would cost between 72p and £1.44; probably nearer the upper figure – say £1.30 as a guess.

Our guess (£1.30) was close to the correct answer (£1.20) – so we can be confident in the calculated answer.

The above is a lengthy way of doing a simple calculation. In reality, we would have completed the calculation in three steps:

$$12 \text{ apples cost £2.88}$$

$$1 \text{ apple cost} \frac{£2.88}{12}$$

$$5 \text{ apples cost} \frac{£2.88}{12} \times 5 = £1.20$$

CHECKING YOUR ANSWER – DOES IT SEEM REASONABLE?

As we have noted, it is good practice to have a rough idea of the answer first, so you can check your final calculated answer. Your estimation can be a single value or, more usually, a range within which your answer should be. If the answer you get is outside this range, then your answer is wrong and you should recheck your calculations.

The following guide may be useful in helping you to decide if your answer is reasonable. Any answer outside these ranges probably means that you have calculated the wrong answer.

The maximum you should give a patient:

Tablets	Not more than 4 for any one dose*
Liquids	Anything from 5 to 20 mL for any one dose
Injections	Anything from 1 to 10 mL for any one dose

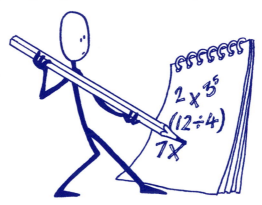

PUTTING IT ALL TOGETHER

Using all the above principles, consider the following situation: You have an injection of pethidine with the strength of 100 mg/2 mL and you need to give a dose of 60 mg.

First – have a rough idea of your answer by estimation. By looking at what you have – 100 mg in 2 mL – you can assume the following:

- The dose you want (60 mg) will be
  - less than 2 mL (2 mL = 100 mg)
  - more than 1 mL (1 mL = 50 mg – by halving)
- 100 mg – 2 mL
- 10 mg – 0.2 mL (by dividing by 10)
- 60 mg – 1.2 mL (by multiplying by 6)
- 200 mg – 2 mL (by doubling)

Although we have calculated the volume required, it is always a good idea to do the calculation to check that you have the right answer.

---

* An exception to this would be prednisolone. Some doses of prednisolone may mean the patient taking up to 10 tablets at any one time. Even with prednisolone, it is important to check the dose and the number of tablets.

Now we can attempt the calculation.
Calculate from first principles – using the 'one unit' rule:

$$100 \text{ mg} = 2 \text{ mL}$$

$$1 \text{ mg} = \frac{2}{100} \text{ mL}$$

$$60 \text{ mg} = \frac{2}{100} \times 60 = 1.2 \text{ mL}$$

Working from first principles, we have arrived at an answer of 1.2 mL. Checking the calculated answer of 1.2 mL with our estimate of 1.2 mL means that we should be confident that our calculated answer is correct.

Does your answer seem reasonable? The answer is yes. It correlates to your estimation and only a part of the ampoule will be used which, from common sense, seems reasonable.

MINIMIZING ERRORS

- Write out the calculation clearly. It is easy to end up reading from the wrong line.
- If you are copying formulas from a reference source, double-check what you have written down.
- Write down every step.
- Remember to include the units at every step; this will avoid any confusion as to what your answer actually means.
- Do not take short cuts; you are more likely to make a mistake.
- Try not to be totally dependent on your calculator. Have an approximate idea of what the answer should be. Then, if you happen to hit the wrong button on the calculator you are more likely to be aware that an error has been made.
- Finally, always double-check your calculation. There is frequently more than one way of doing a calculation, so if you get the same answer by two different methods the chances are that your answer will be correct. Alternatively, try working it in reverse and see if you get the numbers you started with.

REMEMBER

If you are in any doubt about a calculation you are asked to do on the ward, stop and get help.

3 PER CENT AND PERCENTAGES

OBJECTIVES

At the end of this chapter, you should be familiar with the following:

- Per cent and percentages
- Converting fractions to percentages
- Converting percentages to fractions
- Converting decimals to percentages
- Converting percentages to decimals
- Calculations involving percentages
  - How to find the percentage of a number
  - How to find what percentage one number is of another
- Drug calculations involving percentages
- How to use the per cent key on your calculator

KEY POINTS

Per cent

- Per cent means 'part of a hundred' or 'a proportion of a hundred'.
- The symbol for per cent is %, so 30% means 30 parts or units of a hundred.
- Per cent is often used to give a quick indication of a specific quantity and is useful when making comparisons.

Percentages and fractions

- To convert a **fraction** to a **percentage**, **multiply** by 100.
- To convert a **percentage** to a **fraction**, **divide** by 100.

Percentages and decimals

- To convert a **decimal** to a **percentage**, **multiply** by 100 – move the decimal point **two** places to the right.
- To convert a **percentage** to a **decimal**, **divide** by 100 – move the decimal point **two** places to the left.

Knowing approximate conversion for percentages is useful for estimation of answers.

10% = $^1/_{10}$ (one-tenth)
20% = $^2/_{10}$ (two-tenths) or $^1/_5$ (one-fifth)
25% = $^1/_4$ (one-quarter)
30% = $^3/_{10}$ (three-tenths) or $^1/_3$ (one-third)
40% = $^4/_{10}$ (four-tenths) or $^2/_5$ (two-fifths)
50% = $^5/_{10}$ (five-tenths) or $^1/_2$ (half)
60% = $^6/_{10}$ (six-tenths) or $^3/_5$ (three-fifths)
70% = $^7/_{10}$ (seven-tenths) or $^2/_3$ (two-thirds)
75% = $^3/_4$ (three-quarters)
80% = $^8/_{10}$ (eight-tenths) or $^4/_5$ (four-fifths)
90% = $^9/_{10}$ (nine-tenths) or just under one

To find the percentages of a number, always **divide** by 100:

$$\frac{\text{whole}}{100} \times \text{part}$$

To find what percentage one number is of another, always **multiply** by 100%:

$$\frac{\text{part}}{\text{whole}} \times 100$$

INTRODUCTION

The per cent or percentage is a common way of expressing the amount of something and is useful for comparing different quantities.

It is unlikely that you will need to calculate the percentage of something on the ward. It is more likely that you will need to know how much drug is in a solution given as a percentage, e.g. an infusion containing potassium 0.3%.

PER CENT AND PERCENTAGES

As previously noted, a convenient way of expressing drug strengths is by using the per cent. We will be dealing with how percentages are used to describe drug strengths or concentrations in Chapter 6.

The aim of this chapter is to explain the concept of per cent and show how to do simple percentage calculations. It is important to understand per cent before moving on to percentage concentrations.

Per cent (%) means 'part of a hundred' or a 'proportion of a hundred'. So 30% means 30 parts or units of a hundred. The word *per cent* comes from the Latin *per centum*; the Latin word *centum* means 100 – for example, a century is 100 years.

Percentages are often used to give a quick indication of a specific quantity and are useful when making comparisons. For instance, if you consider a town where 5,690 people live and the unemployment numbers are 853, it is very difficult to visualize the proportion of people who are unemployed. It is much easier to say that in a town of 5,690 people, 15% of them are unemployed.

If we consider another town of 11,230 people where 2,246 people are unemployed, it is very difficult to see at a glance which town has the greater proportion of unemployed. When the numbers are given as percentages, it is easier to compare: the first town has 15% unemployment and the second town has 20% unemployed.

Percentages can be useful, and so is being able to convert to a percentage. Numbers or quantities are easier to compare when given as percentages.

CONVERTING FRACTIONS TO PERCENTAGES AND VICE VERSA

To convert a fraction to a percentage, **multiply** by 100:

$$\frac{2}{5} = \frac{2}{5} \times 100 = 40\%$$

To convert a percentage to a fraction, **divide** by 100:

$$40\% = \frac{40}{100} = \frac{4}{10} = \frac{2}{5}$$

If possible, always reduce the fraction to its lowest terms before making the conversion.

CONVERTING DECIMALS TO PERCENTAGES AND VICE VERSA

To convert a decimal to a percentage, once again **multiply** by 100:

$$0.4 = 0.4 \times 100 = 40\%$$

Remember, to multiply by 100, you move the decimal point **two** places to the **right**.

To convert a percentage to a decimal, **divide** by 100:

$$40\% = \frac{40}{100} = 0.4$$

To divide by 100, move the decimal point **two** places to the **left**.

So, to convert fractions and decimals to percentages or vice versa, simply multiply or divide by 100. Thus:

$$25\% = \frac{25}{100} = \frac{1}{4} = 0.25 \text{ (a quarter)}$$

$$0.5 = 0.5 \times 100 = 50\% \text{ (a half)}$$

$$\frac{3}{4} = \frac{3}{4} \times 100 = 75\% \text{ (three-quarters)}$$

Knowing approximate conversion for percentages is useful for estimation of answers:

$10\% = {}^{1}/_{10}$ (one-tenth)

$20\% = {}^{2}/_{10}$ (two-tenths) or ${}^{1}/_{5}$ (one-fifth)

$25\% = {}^{1}/_{4}$ (one-quarter)

$30\% = {}^{3}/_{10}$ (three-tenths) or ${}^{1}/_{3}$ (one-third)

$40\% = {}^{4}/_{10}$ (four-tenths) or ${}^{2}/_{5}$ (two-fifths)

$50\% = {}^{5}/_{10}$ (five-tenths) or ${}^{1}/_{2}$ (a half)

$60\% = {}^{6}/_{10}$ (six-tenths) or ${}^{3}/_{5}$ (three-fifths)

$70\% = {}^{7}/_{10}$ (seven-tenths) or ${}^{2}/_{3}$ (two-thirds)

$75\% = {}^{3}/_{4}$ (three-quarters)

$80\% = {}^{8}/_{10}$ (eight-tenths) or ${}^{4}/_{5}$ (four-fifths)

$90\% = {}^{9}/_{10}$ (nine-tenths) or just under one

The next step is to look at how to find the percentage of something. The following worked example should show how this is done.

CALCULATIONS INVOLVING PERCENTAGES

The first type of calculation we are going to look at is how to find the percentage of a given quantity or number.

WORKED EXAMPLE

How much is 28% of 250?

With this method you are working in percentages. Before attempting the calculation, first estimate the answer.

We can round up the percentage to 30 which we can consider to be approximately one-third. To make the estimation easier, we will round down the number to 240. So we are now looking at one-third of 240, which is 80.

Alternatively, we can estimate the answer by manipulation of numbers. Round up the percentage to 30%:

100% – 250

10% – 25 (by dividing by 10)

30% – 75 (by multiplying by 3)

As the percentage was rounded up, then the answer will be slightly lower – 72 would be a good guess.

Now we can attempt the calculation.

STEP ONE

When doing percentage calculations, the number or quantity you want to find the percentage of is always equal to 100%.

In this example, 250 is equal to 100% and you want to find out how much 28% is. So,

$$250 = 100\%$$

(Thus you are converting the number to a percentage.)

STEP TWO

Calculate how much is equal to 1%, i.e. divide by 100 (you are using the *one unit* rule) – see *First Principles* for an explanation.

$$1\% = \frac{250}{100}$$

STEP THREE

Multiply by the percentage required, (28%):

$$28\% = \frac{250}{100} \times 28 = 70$$

Checking the calculated answer of 70 with our estimation of 72 to 80 means that we should be confident in our calculated answer.

ANSWER: 28% of 250 = 70

We can devise a simple formula:

Per cent means 'part of a hundred', so simply divide the number (whole) by 100, and then multiply by the percentage wanted. This will give us:

$$part = \frac{whole}{100} \times percent$$

In this example:

$$Whole = 250$$

$$Part = 28$$

Substitute the numbers in the formula:

$$\frac{250}{100} \times 28 = 70$$

ANSWER: 28% of 250 = 70

TIP BOX

Whatever method you use, always divide by 100.

However, you may want to find out what percentage a number is of another larger number, especially when comparing numbers or quantities. So this is the second type of percentage calculation we are going to look at.

WORKED EXAMPLE

What percentage is 630 of 9,000?

As before, it is best to work in percentages since it is that you want to find.

Before starting the calculation, we will try and estimate the answer. We can round down 630 to 600 and leave 9,000 as it is:

$$9,000 \quad - \quad 100\%$$

$$900 \quad - \quad 10\% \qquad \text{(dividing by 10)}$$

$$300 \quad - \quad \frac{10}{3} \qquad \text{(dividing by 3)}$$

$$600 \quad - \quad \frac{10}{3} \times 2 \quad \text{(multiplying by 2)}$$

This gives us 20/3 which is approximately just over 6 and under 7. Our estimation would be 6% to 7%. Now we can attempt the calculation.

STEP ONE

Once again, the number or quantity you want to find the percentage of is always equal to 100%.

In this example, 9,000 would be equal to 100% and you want to find out the percentage of 630. So,

$$9,000 = 100\%$$

(Thus you are converting the number to a percentage.)

STEP TWO

Calculate the percentage for 1, i.e. divide by 9,000 using the one unit rule:

$$1 = \frac{100}{9,000}\%$$

STEP THREE

Multiply by the number you wish to find the percentage for, i.e. the smaller number (630):

$$\frac{100}{9,000} \times 630 = 7\%$$

Checking the calculated answer of 7% with our estimation of 6% to 7% means that we should be confident in our calculated answer.

ANSWER: 630 is 7% of 9,000.

Once again, we can devise a simple formula:

Remember, the larger number will be the **whole** and the smaller number will be the **part**, i.e. we will have a fraction – part/whole. To convert a fraction to a percentage, we would multiply by 100. This would give us:

$$\text{per cent} = \frac{\text{part}}{\text{whole}} \times 100$$

In this example:

$$\text{Part} = 630$$

$$\text{Whole} = 9,000$$

Substitute the numbers in the formula:

$$\frac{630}{9,000} \times 100 = 7\%$$

ANSWER: 630 is 7% of 9,000.

TIP BOX

In this case, **multiply** by 100 (it is always on the top line).

DRUG CALCULATIONS INVOLVING PERCENTAGES

The principles here can easily be applied to drug calculations. As before, it is unlikely that you will need to find the percentage of something, but these calculations are included here in order to provide an understanding of per cent and percentages, especially where drugs are concerned. Once again, always convert everything to the same units before solving the calculation.

> **WORKED EXAMPLE**
>
> What volume (in mL) is 60% of 1.25 litres?
>
> Before attempting the calculation, first estimate the answer.
>
> As the volume required and what we have are in different units, convert to the same units (convert litres to millilitres) (please refer to Chapter 4 for further discussion on converting units):
>
> $$1.25 \text{ litres} = 1.25 \times 1,000 = 1,250 \text{ mL}$$
>
> Before starting the calculation, we will try and estimate the answer. We can leave the percentage at 60 which we can consider to be six-tenths. So, we are now looking at sixth-tenths of 1,250 which is:
>
> $$\frac{1,250}{10} \times 6 = 125 \times 6 = 750 \text{ mL}$$
>
> We can make the above easier to calculate by multiplying 125 by 2 (= 250) and adding three lots together (250 + 250 + 250) to give 750.
>
> Alternatively, we can estimate the answer by manipulation of numbers:
>
> | 100% | – | 1,250 mL | |
> |---|---|---|---|
> | 10% | – | 125 mL | (by dividing by 10) |
> | 20% | – | 250 mL | (by multiplying by 2) |
> | 60% | – | 750 mL | (by multiplying by 3) |
>
> Although we have calculated the volume for the percentage, it is always a good idea to do the calculation to check that you have the right answer.
>
> Work in the same units – in this case, work in millilitres as these are the units of the answer:
>
> $$1.25 \text{ litres} = 1.25 \times 1,000 = 1,250 \text{ mL}$$

Remember, the number or quantity you want to find the percentage of is always equal to 100%:

$$1{,}250 \text{ mL} = 100\%$$

(You are converting the volume to a percentage.)
    Thus,

$$1\% = \frac{1{,}250}{100}$$

$$60\% = \frac{1{,}250}{100} \times 60 = 750 \text{ mL}$$

Checking the calculated answer of 750 mL with our estimation of 750 mL means that we should be confident in our calculated answer.

ANSWER: 60% of 1.25 litres equals 750 mL.

Alternatively, you can use the formula:

$$\text{per cent} = \frac{\text{whole}}{100} \times \text{part}$$

Rewriting it as:

$$\frac{\text{what you've got}}{100} \times \text{percentage required}$$

where:
    what you've got = 1,250 mL
    percentage required = 60%

Substitute the numbers in the formula:

$$\frac{1{,}250}{100} \times 60 = 750 \text{ mL}$$

ANSWER: 60% of 1.25 litres is 750 mL.

Now consider the following example.

WORKED EXAMPLE

What percentage is 125 mg of 500 mg?

Before attempting the calculation, first estimate the answer.
    Everything is already in the same units, milligrams (mg), so there is no need for any conversions.
    Looking at the numbers involved, it should be easy to spot that 125 is a quarter of 500. We know that a quarter is equal to 25%.

Alternatively, we can estimate the answer by manipulation of numbers:

$$500 \text{ mg} - 100\%$$

$$250 \text{ mg} - 50\% \quad \text{(by halving)}$$

$$125 \text{ mg} - 25\% \quad \text{(by halving)}$$

Although we have calculated the percentage, it is always a good idea to do the calculation to check that you have the right answer.

Everything is already in the same units, milligrams (mg), so there is no need for any conversions.

As always, the quantity you want to find the percentage of is equal to 100%, i.e.

$$500 \text{ mg} = 100\%$$

(You are converting the amount to a percentage.)

Thus,

$$1 \text{ mg} = \frac{100}{500} \%$$

$$125 \text{ mg} = \frac{100}{500} \times 125 = 25\%$$

Checking the calculated answer of 25% with our estimation of 25% means that we should be confident in our *calculated answer.*

ANSWER: 125 mg is equal to 25% of 500 mg.

Alternatively, you can use the formula:

$$\text{per cent} = \frac{\text{part}}{\text{whole}} \times 100$$

where:

  part = 125 mg
  whole = 500 mg

Substitute the numbers in the formula:

$$\frac{100}{500} \times 125 = 25\%$$

ANSWER: 125 mg is equal to 25% of 500 mg.

HOW TO USE THE PER CENT KEY ON YOUR CALCULATOR

Basic calculators are designed for everyday use and the per cent key [%] is designed as a shortcut so that calculation is not necessary. The per cent key [%] should be considered as a function and not as an operation such as add, subtract, multiply, or divide.

Using the per cent key [%] automatically multiplies by 100. It is also important that the numbers and the per cent key [%] are pressed in the right sequence; otherwise it is quite easy to get the wrong answer.

Not all calculators behave the same way as far as the per cent key is concerned. It is a good idea to experiment with a few simple sums to see how the per cent key works on your own calculator. Alternatively, you can try the following examples.

Let us go back to our original example.

1. How much is 28% of 250?
   You could easily find the answer by the long method, i.e.

$$\frac{250}{100} \times 28$$

Key in the sequence, [2][5][0] [÷] [1][0][0] [×] [2][8] [=], to give an answer of 70. This is exactly the calculation performed by the per cent key [%]. But when using the per cent key [%], you need to enter in the following way:

ENTER	[2][5][0]	DISPLAY = 250
ENTER	[×]	DISPLAY = 250
ENTER	[2][8]	DISPLAY = 28
ENTER	[%]	DISPLAY = 70 (Answer)

Most calculators will give the correct answer (70) without having to press the [=] key. Press the [=] key to see what will happen – it may give an answer of 17,500. If you do get an answer of 17,500, what is probably happening is that by pressing the [=] key, you are multiplying 250 by 28% of 250 (i.e. by the answer):

250 × 28% of 250 *or* 250 × 70 = 17500 (giving a nonsensical answer)

You should realize that the answer is going to be less than 250 (approximately one-third).

REMEMBER

Pressing the per cent key [%] finishes the current calculation. Thus, when using your calculator, *do not press the [=] key.*

Let us now look at the second worked example.

2. What percentage is 630 of 9,000?
   Once again, you can easily find the answer by

$$\frac{630}{9,000} \times 100$$

Key in the sequence [6][3][0] [÷] [9][0][0][0] [×] [1][0][0] [=] to give an answer of 7%.

But when using the per cent key, you need to enter in the following way:

ENTER	[6][3][0]	DISPLAY = 630
ENTER	[÷]	DISPLAY = 630
ENTER	[9][0][0][0]	DISPLAY = 9000
ENTER	[%]	DISPLAY = 7% (answer)

Don't forget, most calculators will give the correct answer (7) without having to press the [=] key,

Once again, pressing the [=] key may give the wrong answer.

What happens is that by pressing the [=] key, you are dividing by 9,000 again, i.e.

$$\frac{630}{9,000 \times 9,000} \times 100$$

You should realize that the answer is going to be less than 10%. Round the numbers up and down to give an easy sum – 600 and 10,000 or 6 and 100 or 6%.

Remember that it is 630 **divided by** 9,000, and not the other way round.

Therefore it is important to enter the numbers the right way round on your calculator.

If you can't remember which way round to enter the numbers, an easy way to remember is enter the **smaller number** (i.e. the **amount**) first.

Also remember, *pressing the per cent key [%] finishes the current calculation.*

Thus, when using your calculator, *do not press the [=] key.*

To summarize, if you want to use the per cent key on your calculator, remember the following:

1. Enter the numbers in the right sequence.

 If you are finding the percentage of something: *multiply* the two numbers. (It doesn't matter in which order you enter the numbers.)

 If you are finding the percentage one number is of another: *divide* the *smaller* number (enter first) by the *larger* number (enter second).

 In this case, the sequence of numbers is important.
2. Always enter or press the [%] key *last*.
3. Do *not* enter or press the [=] key.
4. Refer to your calculator manual to see how your own calculator uses the [%] key.
5. Don't forget to clear your calculator, otherwise the numbers left in your calculator may be carried over to your next sum.

Although using the [%] key is a quick way of finding percentages, you have to use it properly, therefore it may be best to ignore it and do the calculations the long way.

TIP BOX

Get to know how to use your calculator – read the manual. If you don't know how to use your calculator properly, there is the potential for errors. You won't know if the answer you've got is correct or not.

PROBLEMS

Work out the following:

Question 1   30% of 3,090

Question 2   84% of 42,825

Question 3   56.25% of 800

Question 4   60% of 80.6

Question 5   A 10-year-old can be administered 60% of the adult dose. If the adult dose of flucloxacillin is 250 mg, how much should the child receive?

What percentage are the following?

Question 6   60 of 750

Question 7   53,865 of 64,125

Question 8   29.61 of 47

Question 9   53.69 of 191.75

Question 10   You are reviewing the ward stock of infusion bags. Due to limited space, space needs to be made to keep a new strength of infusion. In order to do this, the existing stock needs to be reviewed and the least used infusion will be taken off the ward stock list. Of the following, which infusions should be replaced?

	BAGS A	BAGS B	BAGS C	BAGS D
Used/ordered	52/80	54/90	32/50	45/60

Answers can be found in Chapter 15.

4 UNITS AND EQUIVALENCES

OBJECTIVES

At the end of this chapter, you should be familiar with the following:

- SI units
- Prefixes used in clinical medicine
- Equivalences
  - Equivalences of weight
  - Equivalences of volume
  - Equivalences of amount of substance
- Conversion from one unit to another
- Guide to writing units

KEY POINTS

Equivalences of weight

UNIT	SYMBOL	EQUIVALENT	SYMBOL
1 kilogram	kg	1,000 grams	g
1 gram	g	1,000 milligrams	mg
1 milligram	mg	1,000 micrograms	mcg
1 microgram	mcg	1,000 nanograms	ng

Equivalences of volume

UNIT	SYMBOL	EQUIVALENT	SYMBOL
1 litre	L or l	1,000 millilitres	mL or ml

Equivalences of amount of substance

UNIT	SYMBOL	EQUIVALENT	SYMBOL
1 mole	mol	1,000 millimoles	mmol
1 millimole	mmol	1,000 micromoles	mcmol

- Milligrams, micrograms, and nanograms should be written in full to avoid confusion.
- Avoid decimals. A decimal point written in the wrong place can mean 10- or even 100-fold errors.

> **Converting units**
> * It is always best to work with the smaller unit to avoid the use of decimals.
> * When converting, the amount remains the same, only the unit changes.
> * Remember to look at the units carefully; converting from one unit to another may involve several steps.
> * To convert from a *larger* unit to a *smaller* unit, *multiply* by 1,000.
> * To convert from a *smaller* unit to a *larger* unit, *divide* by 1,000.

INTRODUCTION

Many different units are used in medicine; for example:

* Drug strengths, e.g. digoxin injection 500 micrograms in 1 mL
* Dosages, e.g. dobutamine 3 mcg/kg/min
* Patient electrolyte levels, e.g. sodium 137 mmol/L

It is important to have a basic knowledge of the units used in medicine and how they are derived.

It is particularly important to have an understanding of the units in which drugs can be prescribed and how to convert from one unit to another – this last part is very important as it forms the basis of all drug calculations. In addition, it is possible that you may have to administer a dose prescribed in a different unit to that of the medicines available.

SI UNITS

SI stands for *Système Internationale (d'Unités)* and is another name for the metric system of measurement. The aim of metrication is to make calculations easier than with the imperial system (ounces, pounds, stones, inches, pints, etc.). SI units are generally accepted in the United Kingdom and many other countries for use in medical practice and pharmacy. They were introduced in the NHS in 1975.

SI base units

The main units are those used to measure weight, volume and amount of substance:

* Weight: kilogram (kg)
* Volume: litre (l or L)
* Amount of substance: mole (mol)

SI prefixes

When an SI unit is inconveniently large or small, prefixes are used to denote multiples or submultiples. It is preferable to use multiples of a thousand. For example:

- gram
- milligram (one thousandth, 1/1,000th of a gram)
- microgram (one millionth, 1/1,000,000th of a gram)
- nanogram (one thousand millionth, 1/1,000,000,000th of a gram)

For example, one millionth of a gram could be written as 0.000001 g or as 1 microgram. The second version is easier to read than the first and easier to work with once you understand how to use units and prefixes. It is also less likely to lead to errors, especially when administering drug doses.

PREFIX	SYMBOL	DIVISION/MULTIPLE	FACTOR
Mega	M	× 1,000,000	10^6
Kilo	k	× 1,000	10^3
Deci	d	÷ 10	10^{-1}
Centi	c	÷ 100	10^{-2}
Milli	m	÷ 1,000	10^{-3}
Micro	μ	÷ 1,000,000	10^{-6}
Nano	n	÷ 1,000,000,000	10^{-9}

PREFIXES USED IN CLINICAL PRACTICE

The main prefixes you will come across on the ward are **mega-**, **milli-**, **micro-**, and **nano-**. Thus in practice, drug strengths and dosages can be expressed in various ways:

- Benzylpenicillin is sometimes expressed in terms of mega units (1 mega unit means 1 million units of activity). Each vial contains benzylpenicillin 600 mg, which equals 1 mega unit.
- Small volumes of liquids are often expressed in millilitres (mL) and are used to describe small volumes, e.g. lactulose, 10 mL to be given three times a day.
- Drug strengths are usually expressed in milligrams (mg), e.g. furosemide 40 mg tablets.

- When the amount of drug in a tablet or other formulation is very small, strengths are expressed as micrograms or even nanograms, e.g. digoxin 125 microgram tablets; alfacalcidol 250 nanogram capsules.

EQUIVALENCES

The SI base units are too large for everyday clinical use, so they are subdivided into multiples of 1,000.

Equivalences of weight

UNIT	SYMBOL	EQUIVALENT	SYMBOL
1 kilogram	kg	1,000 grams	g
1 gram	g	1,000 milligrams	mg
1 milligram	mg	1,000 micrograms	mcg
1 nanogram	mcg	1,000 nanograms	ng

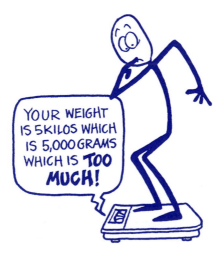

YOUR WEIGHT IS 5 KILOS WHICH IS 5,000 GRAMS WHICH IS **TOO MUCH!**

Equivalences of volume

UNIT	SYMBOL	EQUIVALENT	SYMBOL
1 litre	L or l*	1,000 millilitres	mL or ml

* See notes on *Guide to Writing Units* below.

Equivalences of amount of substance

UNIT	SYMBOL	EQUIVALENT	SYMBOL
1 mole	mol	1,000 millimoles	mmol
1 millimole	mmol	1,000 micromoles	mcmol

Moles and millimoles are the terms used by chemists when measuring quantities of certain substances or chemicals; they are more accurate than using grams. For a more extensive explanation, see Chapter 5.

Examples include:

$$0.5 \text{ kg} = 500 \text{ g}$$
$$0.25 \text{ g} = 250 \text{ mg}$$
$$0.2 \text{ mg} = 200 \text{ mcg}$$
$$0.5 \text{ L} = 500 \text{ mL}$$
$$0.25 \text{ mol} = 250 \text{ mmol}$$

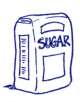

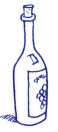

1 Kg
1,000 g
1,000,000 mg
1,000,000,000 mcg
1,000,000,000,000 ng

1 l
1,000 ml

1 mole
1 mol
1,000 mmol
1,000,000 mcmol

CONVERSION FROM ONE UNIT TO ANOTHER

In drug calculations, it is best to work in whole numbers, i.e. 125 micrograms and not 0.125 mg, as fewer mistakes are then made. Avoid using decimals, as the decimal point can be written in the wrong place during calculations. A decimal point in the wrong place can mean errors of 10-fold or even 100-fold.

It is always best to work with the smaller unit in order to avoid decimals and decimal points, so you need to be able to convert easily from one unit to another. In general:

- To convert form a **larger** unit to a **smaller** unit, **multiply** by multiples of 1,000.
- To convert from a **smaller** unit to a **larger** unit, **divide** by multiples of 1,000.

For each multiplication or division by 1,000, the decimal point moves three places either to the right or left, depending upon whether you are converting from a larger unit to a smaller unit or vice versa.

Wright (2009) suggests a technique for remembering whether to multiply or divide by 1,000 when converting units. If you consider whether the unit you are converting to is heavier or lighter than the original, this will guide you. Take for example milligrams to grams. Grams are heavier than milligrams, so you need 'less weight' and hence the number will get smaller – *divide*. Conversely, if you are converting from grams to milligrams, milligrams are 'lighter', so then more of them are needed – *multiply*.

When you have to convert from a very large unit to a much smaller unit (or vice versa), you may find it easier to do the conversion in several steps.

For example, to convert 0.005 kg to milligrams, first convert to grams:

$$0.005 \text{ kg} = 0.005 \times 1,000 = 5 \text{ g}$$

Next, convert grams to milligrams:

$$5 \text{ g} = 5 \times 1,000 = 5,000 \text{ mg}$$

REMEMBER

When you do conversions like this, the amount remains the same; it is only the units that change. Obviously, it appears more when expressed as a smaller unit, but the **amount remains the same** (200 pence is the same as £2, although it may look more).

Reference

Wright K. Developing methods for solving drug dosage calculations. *British Journal of Nursing* 2009; 18(11): 685–689.

WORKED EXAMPLES

EXAMPLE ONE

Convert 0.5 g to milligrams.

You are going from a larger unit to a smaller unit, so you have to multiply by 1,000:

$$0.5 \text{ g} \times 1,000 = 500 \text{ milligrams}$$

The decimal point moves three places to the right.

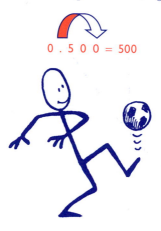

0 . 5 0 0 = 500

EXAMPLE TWO

Convert 2,000 g to kilograms.

You are going from a smaller unit to a larger unit, so you have to divide by 1,000:

$$2,000 \text{ g} = \frac{2,000}{1,000} = 2 \text{ kg}$$

The decimal point moves three places to the left.

2 0 0 0 . = 2

EXAMPLE THREE

Convert 150 nanograms to micrograms.

You are going from a smaller unit to a larger unit, so you have to divide by 1,000:

$$\frac{150}{1,000} \text{ nanograms} = 0.150 \text{ micrograms}$$

The decimal point moves three places to the left.

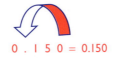

0 . 1 5 0 = 0.150

GUIDE TO WRITING UNITS

The *British National Formulary* makes the following recommendations:

- The unnecessary use of decimal points should be avoided, e.g. 3 mg, *not* 3.0 mg.
- Quantities of 1 gram or more should be expressed as 1.5 g, etc.
- Quantities less than 1 gram should be written in milligrams, e.g. 500 mg, *not* 0.5 g.
- Quantities less than 1 mg should be written in micrograms, e.g. 100 micrograms, *not* 0.1 mg.
- When decimals are unavoidable, a zero should be written in front of the decimal point where there is no other figure, e.g. 0.5 mL *not* .5 mL.
- However, the use of a decimal point is acceptable to express a range, e.g. 0.5–1 g.
- Micrograms and nanograms should *not* be abbreviated. Similarly, the word 'units' should *not* be abbreviated.
- A capital L is used for litre, to avoid confusion (a small l could be mistaken for a figure 1, especially when typed or printed).
- Cubic centimetre, or cm^3 is *not* used in medicine or pharmacy; use millilitre (mL or ml) instead.

The following two case reports illustrate examples where bad writing can lead to problems.

CONFUSING MICROGRAMS AND MILLIGRAMS

Case report

On admission to hospital, a patient taking thyroxine replacement therapy presented her general practitioner's referral letter which stated that her maintenance dose was 0.025 mg once daily. The clerking house officer incorrectly converted this dose and prescribed 250 micrograms rather than the 25 micrograms required. A dose was administered before the error was detected by the ward pharmacist the next morning.

From *Pharmacy in Practice* 1994;4: 124.

This example highlights several errors:

- The wrong units were originally used – milligrams instead of micrograms.
- A number containing a decimal point was used.
- Conversion from one unit to another was incorrectly carried out.

THIS UNIT ABBREVIATION IS DANGEROUS

Case report

Patient received 50 units of insulin instead of the prescribed STAT dose of 5 units. A junior doctor requiring a patient to be given a STAT dose of 5 units Actrapid insulin wrote the prescription appropriately but chose to incorporate the abbreviation ⊙ for 'units' that occasionally is used on written requests for units of blood. Thus the prescription read: 'Actrapid insulin 5 ⊙ STAT'.

The administering nurse misread the abbreviation used and interpreted the prescription as 50 units of insulin. This was administered to the patient who of course became profoundly hypoglycaemic and required urgent medical intervention.

Comment

The use of the symbol ⊙ to indicate units of blood is an old-fashioned practice which is now in decline. This case serves to illustrate the catastrophic effect that the inappropriate use of this abbreviation can have – it led to misinterpretation by the nursing staff and resulted in harm to the patient.

From *Pharmacy in Practice* 1995;5: 131.

This example illustrates that abbreviations should not be used. As recommended, the word 'units' should *not* be abbreviated.

PROBLEMS

Work out the following:

Question 1   Convert 0.0125 kilograms to grams.

Question 2   Convert 250 nanograms to micrograms.

Question 3   Convert 3.2 litres to millilitres.

Question 4   Convert 0.0273 moles to millimoles.

Question 5   Convert 3,750 grams to kilograms.

Question 6   Convert 0.05 grams to micrograms.

Question 7   Convert 25,000 milligrams to kilograms.

Question 8   Convert 4.5×10^{-6} grams to nanograms.

Question 9   You have an ampoule of digoxin 0.25 mg/mL. Calculate the amount (in micrograms) in a 2 mL ampoule.

Question 10   You have an ampoule of fentanyl 0.05 mg/mL. Calculate the amount (in micrograms) in a 2 mL ampoule.

Answers can be found in Chapter 15.

5 MOLES AND MILLIMOLES

OBJECTIVES

At the end of this chapter, you should be familiar with the following:

- Moles and millimoles
- Calculations involving moles and millimoles
- Conversion of milligrams to millimoles
- Conversion of percentage strength (% w/v) to millimoles

KEY POINTS

Moles

- The *mole* is a unit used by chemists to count atoms and molecules.
- A *mole* of any substance is the amount which contains the same number of particles of the substance as there are atoms in 12 g of carbon (C12) – known as Avogadro's number.
- For elements or atoms:

  one mole = the *atomic mass* in grams
- For molecules:

  one mole = the *molecular mass* in grams

Millimoles

- Moles are too big for everyday use, so the unit millimoles is used.
- One millimole is equal to one-thousandth of a mole.
- If one mole is the atomic mass or molecular mass in grams, then it follows that:

  one *millimole* = the *atomic mass* or *molecular mass* in *milligrams*

Conversion of milligrams (mg/mL) to millimoles (mmol)

$$\text{total number of millimoles} = \frac{\text{mg/mL}}{\text{mg of substance containing 1 mmol}} \times \text{volume (in mL)}$$

Conversion of percentage strength (% w/v) to millimoles

$$\text{total number of mmol} = \frac{\text{percentage strength (\% w/v)}}{\text{mg of substance containing 1 mmol}} \times 10 \times \text{volume (mL)}$$

INTRODUCTION

Daily references may be made to moles and millimoles in relation to electrolyte levels, blood glucose, serum creatinine, or other blood results with regard to patients. These are measurements carried out by chemical pathology and the units used are usually millimoles or micromoles. The unit millimole is also encountered with infusions when electrolytes have been added.

For example:

Mr J. Brown   Sodium = 138 mmol/L

'An infusion contains 20 mmol potassium chloride.'

Before you can interpret such results or amounts, you will need to be familiar with this rather confusing unit: the mole. This section will explain what moles and millimoles are and how to do calculations involving millimoles.

WHAT ARE MOLES AND MILLIMOLES?

It is important to know what moles and millimoles are and how they are derived. However, the concept of moles and millimoles is difficult to explain and to understand unless you are familiar with basic chemistry.

Chemists are concerned with atoms, ions, and molecules. These are too small to be counted individually, so the mole is the unit used by chemists to make counting and measuring easier.

So what is a mole? Just as the word *dozen* represents the number 12, the mole also represents a number: 6×10^{23}. This number can represent atoms, ions, or molecules, e.g. 1 mole of atoms is 6×10^{23} atoms. The mole is the SI unit for the amount of a substance, and so one mole is the relative atomic mass or molecular mass in grams. The values of these are given in scientific tables.

The relative atomic mass of potassium is 39; so 1 mole of potassium has a mass of 39 g (which is the same as saying 6×10^{23} atoms of potassium has a mass of 39 g).

Similarly, the molecular mass of sodium chloride is 58.5, therefore a mole of sodium chloride weighs 58.5 g and so 2 moles of sodium chloride weigh 117 g (2×58.5).

Chemists are not the only people who count by weighing. Bank clerks use the same idea when they count coins by weighing them. For example, one hundred 1p coins weigh 356 g; so it is quicker to weigh 356 g of 1p coins than to count a hundred coins.

Now consider a molecule of sodium chloride (NaCl) which consists of one sodium ion (Na^+) and one chloride ion (Cl^-):

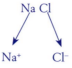

Since moles can refer to atoms as well as molecules, it can be seen that one mole of sodium chloride contains one mole of sodium and one mole of chloride.

Next consider calcium chloride ($CaCl_2$).

It consists of *one* calcium ion and *two* chloride ions.

The '2' after the 'Cl' means *two* lots of chloride:

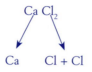

Since moles can refer to atoms as well as molecules, it can be seen that one mole of calcium chloride contains one mole of calcium and two moles of chloride.

Now the molecular mass of calcium chloride is 147 g and not 111 g as expected (by adding the values for $1 \times Ca$ and $2 \times Cl$). The reason for this is that, sometimes, water forms a part of the molecule.

It is actually $CaCl_2 \cdot 2H_2O$, and so 1 mole weighs 147 g. However, from the molecular formula and knowledge of the atomic weights, it can be seen that calcium chloride contains:

I mole of Ca = 40 g
2 moles of Cl = 71 g
2 moles of H_2O, each mole of water = 18 g; $2 \times 18 = 36$ g

So adding everything together:

$$(40 + 71 + 36) = 147 \text{ g}$$

MILLIMOLES AND MICROMOLES

Moles are too big for everyday use, so millimoles and micromoles are used.

One millimole is equal to
one-thousandth of a mole
One micromole is equal to
one-thousandth of a millimole

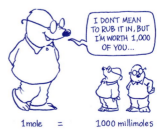

Then it follows that:

I mole contains 1,000 millimoles (mmol)

I millimole contains 1,000 micromoles (mcmol)

If moles are expressed in terms of grams, then it follows that:

I millimole is expressed in terms of milligrams

I micromole is expressed in terms of micrograms

So:

Sodium chloride	would give →	sodium	+	chloride
I mole or I millimole		I mole or I millimole		I mole or I millimole
58.5 g or 58.5 mg		23 g or 23 mg		35.5 g or 35.5 mg

The following are examples and problems to test your understanding of the concept of millimoles. It is unlikely that you will encounter these types of calculations on the ward, but it is useful to know how they are done and can be used for reference if necessary.

The first example converts a mg/mL strength to millimoles.

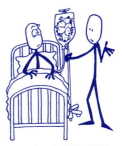

WELL, YES... THE DRUG CHART **DID** SAY 100 millimoles / litre BUT I COULD ONLY SQUEEZE IN 10!

WORKED EXAMPLE

How many millimoles of sodium are there in a 500 mL infusion containing 1.8 mg/mL sodium chloride? From tables, the molecular mass of sodium chloride (NaCl) = 58.5.

Before attempting the calculation, first estimate the answer.

As noted, 1 millimole of sodium chloride yields 1 millimole of sodium, so it follows that the amount (in milligrams) equal to 1 millimole of sodium chloride will give 1 millimole of sodium.

We have 1.8 mg/mL sodium chloride – to make the calculation easier, round up to 2 mg/mL. So:

500 mL = 500 × 2 = 1,000 mg

From tables, the molecular mass of sodium chloride (NaCl) = 58.5; for ease of calculation, round up to 60 (i.e. 1 mmol = 60 mg).

It follows:

$$1 \, mg = \frac{1}{60}$$

$$1,000 \, mg = \frac{1}{60} \times 1,000 = \frac{100}{6}$$

which is approximately equal to $\frac{96}{6} = 16$ mmol.

As the strength of the infusion and the amount for 1 mmol has been increased, 16 mmol is a good guess.

Now we can attempt the calculation.

STEP ONE

As noted, 1 millimole of sodium chloride yields 1 millimole of sodium, so it follows that the amount (in milligrams) equal to 1 millimole of sodium chloride will give 1 millimole of sodium.

In this case, calculate the total amount (in milligrams) of sodium chloride and convert this to millimoles to find out the number of millimoles of sodium.

STEP TWO

Calculate the total amount of sodium chloride.

You have an infusion containing 1.8 mg/mL.

Therefore in 500 mL, you have:

$$1.8 \times 500 = 900 \text{ mg sodium chloride}$$

STEP THREE

From tables, the molecular mass of sodium chloride (NaCl) = 58.5.

So 1 millimole of sodium chloride (NaCl) will weigh 58.5 mg and this amount will give 1 millimole of sodium (Na).

STEP FOUR

Next calculate the number of millimoles in the infusion. First work out the number of millimoles for 1 mg of sodium chloride, then the number for the total amount.

58.5 mg sodium chloride will give 1 millimole of sodium.

$$1 \text{ mg will give } \frac{1}{58.5} \text{ millimoles of sodium}$$

So, $900 \text{ mg will give } \frac{1}{58.5} \times 900 = 15.38 \text{ mmol (or 15.4 mmol [rounding up])}$

Checking the calculated answer of 15.4 mmol with our estimate of 16 mmol means that we should be confident that our calculated answer is correct.

ANSWER: There are 15.4 mmol (approximately 15 mmol) of sodium in a 500 mL infusion containing 1.8 mg/mL sodium chloride.

Alternatively, a formula can be used:

$$\text{total number of millimoles} = \frac{\text{mg/mL}}{\text{mg of substance containing 1 mmol}} \times \text{volume (mL)}$$

where, in this case:

mg/mL = 1.8
mg of substance containing 1 mmol = 58.5
volume (mL) = 500

Substitute the numbers in the formula:

$$\frac{1.8}{58.5} \times 500 = 15.38 \text{ mmol (or 15.4 mmol [rounding up])}$$

ANSWER: There are 15.4 mmol (approximately 15 mmol) of sodium in a 500 mL infusion containing 1.8 mg/mL sodium chloride.

The next example converts percentage strength to millimoles.

WORKED EXAMPLE

How many millimoles of sodium are in 1 litre of sodium chloride 0.9% infusion?

From tables, the molecular mass of sodium chloride (NaCl) = 58.5.
     Before attempting the calculation, first estimate the answer.
     As stated, 1 millimole of sodium chloride yields 1 millimole of sodium. So it follows that the amount (in milligrams) equal to 1 millimole of sodium chloride will give 1 millimole of sodium (see Chapter 6 for further explanation).

We have 0.9% sodium chloride which is 0.9 g per 100 mL.

So, for 1,000 mL = 0.9 × 10 = 9 g.

Convert grams to milligrams by multiplying by 1,000: 9 × 1,000 = 9,000 mg.

From tables, the molecular mass of sodium chloride (NaCl) = 58.5; for ease of calculation, round up to 60 (i.e. 1 mmol = 60 mg).
     It follows that:

$$1 \text{ mg} = \frac{1}{60}$$

$$9,000 \text{ mg} = \frac{1}{60} \times 9,000 = \frac{900}{6} = 150 \text{ mmol}$$

As the amount for 1 mmol has been rounded up, then the actual answer should be slightly higher – 152 mmol is a good guess.

Now we can attempt the calculation.

STEP ONE

We know that 1 millimole of sodium chloride will give 1 millimole of sodium. So, the amount (in milligrams) equal to 1 millimole of sodium chloride will give 1 millimole of sodium.

STEP TWO

To calculate the number of milligrams in 1 millimole of sodium chloride, either refer to tables or work from first principles using atomic masses.

From tables, the molecular mass of sodium chloride (NaCl) = 58.5.

So 1 millimole of sodium chloride (NaCl) will weigh 58.5 mg and this amount will give 1 millimole of sodium (Na).

STEP THREE

Calculate the total amount of sodium chloride present:

$$0.9\% = 0.9 \text{ g in 100 mL}$$

$$= 900 \text{ mg in 100 mL}$$

Thus for a 1 L (1,000 mL) infusion, the amount equals:

$$\frac{900}{100} \times 1,000 = 9,000 \text{ mg}$$

STEP FOUR

From Step Two, it was found that:

58.5 mg sodium chloride will give 1 millimole of sodium.

So it follows that:

1 mg of sodium chloride will give $\frac{1}{58.5}$ millimoles of sodium.

So:

9,000 mg sodium chloride $= \frac{1}{58.5} \times 9,000 = 153.8 \text{ (154) mmol sodium}$

Checking the calculated answer of 154 mmol with our estimate of 150 mmol means that we should be confident that our calculated answer is correct.

ANSWER: 1 litre of sodium chloride 0.9% infusion contains 154 mmol of sodium (approx.).

A formula can be devised:

$$\frac{\text{total number of}}{\text{mmol}} = \frac{\text{percentage strength (\% w/v)}}{\text{mg of substance containing 1 mmol}} \times 10 \times \text{volume (mL)}$$

where in this case:

Percentage strength (% w/v) = 0.9
mg of substance containing 1 mmol = 58.5
Volume = 1,000

Then 10 simply converts percentage strength (g/100 mL) to mg/mL (everything in the same units).

Substituting the numbers in the formula:

$$\frac{0.9}{58.5} \times 10 \times 1,000 = 153.8 \text{ (154) mmol sodium}$$

ANSWER: 1 litre of sodium chloride 0.9% infusion contains 154 mmol of sodium (approx.).

PROBLEMS

To see if you have understood the concept of moles, you may want to try the following:

Question 1   How many millimoles of sodium are there in a 10 mL ampoule containing 300 mg/mL sodium chloride? (Molecular mass of sodium chloride = 58.5.)

Question 2   How many millimoles of sodium are there in a 200 mL infusion of sodium bicarbonate 8.4%? (Molecular mass of sodium bicarbonate = 84.)

Answers can be found in Chapter 15.

6 DRUG STRENGTHS OR CONCENTRATIONS

OBJECTIVES

At the end of this chapter, you should be familiar with the following:

- Percentage concentration
  - Calculating the total amount of drug in a solution
- mg/mL concentrations
  - Converting percentages to a mg/mL concentration
- 'I in …' concentrations or ratio strengths
- Parts per million (ppm)
- Drug concentrations expressed in units: heparin and insulin

KEY POINTS

Percentage concentration

% w/v = number of grams in 100 mL

(A solid is dissolved in a liquid, thus 5% w/v means 5 g in 100 mL.)

% w/w = number of grams in 100 g

(A solid is mixed with another solid, thus 5% w/w means 5 g in 100 g.)

% v/v = number of mL in 100 mL

(A liquid is mixed or diluted with another liquid, thus 5% v/v means 5 mL in 100 mL.)

- The most common percentage strength encountered is the % w/v.
- There will always be the same amount of drug present in 100 mL irrespective of the total volume. Thus in our earlier example of 5% w/v, there are 5 g dissolved in each 100 mL of fluid and this will remain the same if it is a 500 mL bag or a 1 L bag.
- To find the total amount of drug present, the total volume must be taken into account – there is a total of 25 g present in 500 mL of a 5% w/v solution.

mg/mL concentrations

- Defined as the number of mg of drug per mL of liquid.
- Oral liquids – usually expressed as the number of mg in a standard 5 mL spoonful, e.g. erythromycin 250 mg in 5 mL.
- Injections – usually expressed as the number of mg per volume of the ampoule (1 mL, 2 mL, 5 mL, 10 mL and 20 mL), e.g. gentamicin 80 mg in 2 mL.

Strengths can also be expressed in mcg/mL.

Converting percentage concentrations to mg/mL concentrations
• Multiply the percentage by 10 – lidocaine 0.2% = 2 mg/mL.

Converting mg/mL concentrations to percentage concentrations
• Divide the mg/mL strength by 10 – lidocaine 2 mg/mL = 0.2%.

'I in …' concentrations or ratio strengths
• Defined as: **one** gram in however many mL.

For example:

I in 1,000 means 1 g in 1,000 mL

I in 10,000 means 1 g in 10,000 mL

Parts per million (ppm)
• Similar to ratio strengths, but this is used to describe very dilute concentrations.
• Most common concentration encountered is a solid dissolved in a liquid, but can also apply to two solids or liquids mixed together.
• Defined as: **one** gram in 1,000,000 mL *or* **one** milligram in 1 litre.

Units: heparin and insulin
• The purity of drugs such as heparin and insulin from animal or biosynthetic sources varies.
• Therefore these drugs are expressed in terms of **units** as a standard measurement rather than weight.

INTRODUCTION

There are various ways of expressing how much actual drug is present in a medicine. These medicines are usually liquids that are for oral or parenteral administration, but also include those for topical use.

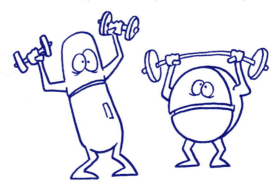

The aim of this chapter is to explain the various ways in which drug strengths can be stated.

PERCENTAGE CONCENTRATION

Following on from the previous chapter, one method of describing concentration is to use the percentage as a unit. Percentage can be defined as the amount of ingredient of drug in 100 parts of the product.

The most common one you will come across is the percentage concentration, w/v (weight in volume). This is when a solid is dissolved in a liquid and means the number of grams dissolved in 100 mL:

> % w/v = number of grams in 100 mL
> (Thus 5% w/v means 5 g in 100 mL.)

Another type of concentration you might come across is the percentage concentration, w/w (weight in weight). This is when a solid is mixed with another solid, e.g. creams and ointments, and means the number of grams in 100 g:

> % w/w = number of grams in 100 g
> (Thus 5% w/w means 5 g in 100 g.)

Another concentration is the percentage concentration, v/v (volume in volume). This is when a liquid is mixed or diluted with another liquid, and means the number of millilitres (mL) in 100 mL:

> % v/v = number of mL in 100 mL
> (Thus 5% v/v means 5 mL in 100 mL.)

The most common percentage concentration you will encounter is the percentage w/v or 'weight in volume' and therefore will be the one considered here.

Thus in our earlier example of 5% w/v, there are 5 g in 100 mL irrespective of the size of the container. For example, glucose 5% infusion means that there are 5 g of glucose dissolved in each 100 mL of fluid, and this will remain the same if it is a 500 mL bag or a 1 L bag.

To find the total amount of drug present in a bottle or infusion bag, you must take into account the size or volume of the bottle or infusion bag.

WORKED EXAMPLE

To calculate the total amount of drug in a solution

How much sodium bicarbonate is there in a 200 mL infusion sodium bicarbonate 8.4% w/v?

STEP ONE

Convert the percentage to the number of grams in 100 mL, i.e.

$$8.4\% \text{ w/v} = 8.4 \text{ g in } 100 \text{ mL}$$

(You are converting the percentage to a specific quantity.)

Before attempting the calculation, first estimate the answer.

By looking at the numbers, we can see that what we want to know is twice that we have written:

$$2 \times 100 = \text{mL} = 8.4 \times 2 = 16.8 \text{ g}$$

Now calculate the answer to check your estimate.

STEP TWO

Calculate how many grams there are in 1 mL, i.e. divide by 100:

$$\frac{8.4}{100} \text{ g in } 1\text{mL}$$

(Use the 'one unit' rule.)

STEP THREE

However, you have a 200 mL infusion. So to find out the total amount present, multiply how much is in 1 mL by the volume you've got (200 mL):

$$\frac{8.4}{100} \times 200 = 16.8 \text{ g in } 200 \text{ mL}$$

ANSWER: There are 16.8 g of sodium bicarbonate in 200 mL of sodium bicarbonate 8.4% w/v infusion.

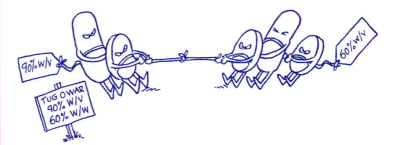

A simple formula can be devised based upon a formula seen earlier:

$$\text{part} = \frac{\text{whole}}{100} \times \text{percent}$$

This can be rewritten as:

$$\text{total amount}\,(g) = \frac{\text{percentage}}{100} \times \text{total volume}\,(mL)$$

Therefore in the worked example:

$$\text{percentage} = 8.4$$

$$\text{total volume (mL)} = 200$$

Substituting the numbers in the formula:

$$\text{total amount}\,(g) = \frac{8.4}{100} \times 200 = 16.8\,g$$

ANSWER: There are 16.8 g of sodium bicarbonate in 200 mL of sodium bicarbonate 8.4% w/v infusion.

PROBLEMS

Calculate how many grams there are in the following:

Question 1   How many grams of sodium chloride are there in a litre infusion of sodium chloride 0.9% w/v?

Question 2   How many grams of potassium, sodium, and glucose are there in a litre infusion of potassium 0.3% w/v, sodium chloride 0.18% w/v, and glucose 4% w/v?

Question 3   How many grams of sodium chloride are there in a 500 mL infusion of sodium chloride 0.45% w/v?

Question 4   You need to give calcium gluconate 2 g as a slow intravenous injection. You have 10 mL ampoules of calcium gluconate 10% w/v. How much do you need to draw up?

Answers can be found in Chapter 15.

mg/mL CONCENTRATIONS

Another way of expressing the amount or concentration of drug in a solution, usually for oral or parenteral administration, is mg/mL, i.e. number of milligrams of drug per mL of liquid. This is the most common way of expressing the amount of drug in a solution.

For oral liquids, it is usually expressed as the number of milligrams in a standard 5 mL spoonful, e.g. amoxicillin 250 mg in 5 mL.

For oral doses that are less than 5 mL an oral syringe would be used, see Chapter 10.

For injections, it is usually expressed as the number of milligrams per volume of the ampoule (1 mL, 2 mL, 5 mL, 10 mL, and 20 mL), e.g. gentamicin 80 mg in 2 mL. However, injections may still be expressed as the number of milligrams per mL, e.g. furosemide 10 mg/mL, 2 mL; particularly in old reference sources.

Note: Strengths can also be expressed in mcg/mL, e.g. hyoscine injection 600 micrograms/1 mL. Only mg/mL will be considered here, but the principles learned here can be applied to other concentrations or strengths, e.g. micrograms/mL. Sometimes it may be useful to convert percentage concentrations to mg/mL concentrations. For example:

lidocaine 0.2%	=	0.2 g per 100 mL
	=	200 mg per 100 mL
	=	2 mg per mL (2 mg/mL)
sodium chloride 0.9%	=	0.9 g per 100 mL
	=	900 mg per 100 mL
	=	9 mg per mL (9 mg/mL)
glucose 5%	=	5 g per 100 mL
	=	5,000 mg per 100 mL
	=	50 mg per mL (50 mg/mL)

This will give the strength of the solution irrespective of the size of the bottle, infusion bag, etc. An easy way of finding the strength in mg/mL is by simply multiplying the percentage by 10. This can be explained using lidocaine 0.2% as an example:

You have lidocaine 0.2% – this is equal to 0.2 g in 100 mL.

Divide by 100 to find out how much is in 1 mL. Thus:

$$\frac{0.2}{100} \text{ g/mL}$$

Multiply by 1,000 to convert grams to milligrams. Thus:

$$\frac{0.2}{100} \times 1,000 \text{ mg/mL}$$

Simplify the above sum to give:

$$0.2 \times 10 = 2 \text{ mg/mL}$$

Therefore you simply multiply the percentage by 10.

With our earlier examples:

Lidocaine 0.2% $= 0.2 \times 10 = 2$ mg/mL

Sodium chloride 0.9% $= 0.9 \times 10 = 9$ mg/mL

Glucose 5% $=\ \ 5 \times 10 = 50$ mg/mL

Conversely, to convert an mg/mL concentration to a percentage, you simply divide by 10.

Once again, if we use our original lidocaine as an example, you have lidocaine 2 mg/mL. Percentage means 'per 100 mL', so multiply by 100, i.e.

2 mg/mL × 100 = 200 mg/100 mL (2 × 100)

Percentage (w/v) means 'the number of grams per 100 mL', so you will have to convert milligrams to grams by dividing by 1,000, i.e.

$$\frac{2 \times 100}{1,000} = \frac{2}{10} = 0.2\%$$

Therefore you simply divide the mg/mL concentration by 10.
With our earlier examples:

Lidocaine 2 mg/mL   = 2 ÷ 10 = 0.2%

Sodium chloride 9 mg/mL   = 9 ÷ 10 = 0.9%

Glucose 50 mg/mL   = 50 ÷ 10 = 5%

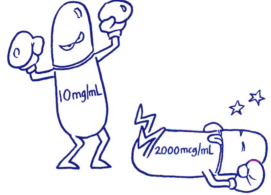

PROBLEMS

Calculate the strengths (mg/mL) for the following:

Question 5   Sodium chloride infusion 0.45% w/v

Question 6   Metronidazole infusion 0.5% w/v

Question 7   Potassium chloride 0.2% w/v, sodium chloride 0.18% w/v, and glucose 4% w/v

Convert the following back to a percentage strength:

Question 8   Bupivacaine 2.5 mg/mL

Question 9   Glucose 500 mg/mL

Question 10   Isosorbide dinitrate 500 micrograms/mL

Answers can be found in Chapter 15.

'I IN ...' CONCENTRATIONS OR RATIO STRENGTHS

This type of concentration is only used occasionally, and is written as '1 in ...' (1 in 10,000), and is sometimes known as a ratio strength. It usually applies to a solid dissolved in a liquid, and by agreed convention the weight is expressed in grams and the volume in millilitres.

So, it means 1 gram in however many mL. For example:

I in 1,000 means I g in 1,000 mL

I in 10,000 means I g in 10,000 mL

Therefore it can be seen that 1 in 10,000 is weaker than 1 in 1,000. So, higher the 'number' the weaker the solution.

The drug most commonly expressed this way is adrenaline/epinephrine:

Adrenaline/epinephrine I in 1,000 which is equal to I mg in I mL

Adrenaline/epinephrine I in 10,000 which is equal to I mg in 10 mL

An easy way to remember the above is to cancel out the three zeroes that appear after the comma, i.e.

Adrenaline/epinephrine I in 1,000 – cancel out the

three zeroes after the comma = 1,0̸0̸0̸ to give:

I in I which can be written as: I mg in I mL

Similarly, for adrenaline/epinephrine 1 in 10,000 – cancel out the three zeroes after the comma to give 10,0̸0̸0̸ to give: 1 in 10 which can be written as: 1 mg in 10 mL.

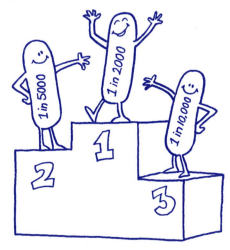

PARTS PER MILLION (ppm)

This is a way of expressing very dilute concentrations. Just as per cent means 'out of a hundred', so parts per million (ppm) means 'out of a million'. It usually applies to a solid dissolved in a liquid, but as with percentage concentrations, it can also apply to two solids or two liquids mixed together.

Once again, by agreed convention:

1 ppm means 1 g in 1,000,000 mL or 1 mg in 1 litre (1,000 mL)

In terms of percentage, 1 ppm equals 0.0001%.
Other equivalents include:

One part per million is one second in 12 days of your life!

One part per million is one penny out of £10,000!

For example, solutions produced by disinfectant chlorine releasing agents are measured in terms of parts per million, such as 1,000 ppm available chlorine.

WORKED EXAMPLE

Sodium hypochlorite solution 2% w/v (20,000 ppm available chloride) needs to be diluted to give a solution containing 125 ppm in 4 litres.

When you are trying to solve these types of problems, it is much easier to work backwards and convert everything to an amount (either in grams or milligrams).

We need 125 ppm in 4 litres – both are in different units; the volume for ppm is millilitres and the volume of the solution is litres. Convert everything to millilitres – so 4 litres equals 4,000 mL.

So 125 ppm means 125 g per 1,000,000 mL or 125 mg in 1,000 mL; so the equivalent for 4,000 mL.

We have: 1,000 mL   –   125 mg
It follows: 4,000 mL   –   500 mg   (multiply by 4)

So, 500 mg in 4,000 mL is the same as 125 ppm.

Next estimate the volume of the concentrated or stock solution equivalent to 500 mg.

Then 20,000 ppm means 20,000 g per 1,000,000 mL or 20,000 mg in 1,000 mL; so the equivalent for 500 mg:

We have: 20,000 mg   –   1,000 mL
So: 1,000 mg   –   50 mL   (divide by 20)
It follows: 500 mg   –   25 mL   (divide by 2).

We need to dilute 25 mL of a 20,000 ppm solution to 4 litres to give a solution of 125 ppm.

Although we have calculated the answer needed, it is always a good idea to do the calculation to check that you have the right answer.

Now we can attempt the calculation.

STEP ONE

Write down the final concentration required:

125 ppm means 125 g per 1,000,000 mL or 125 mg in 1,000 mL.

STEP TWO

Next calculate the amount in 1 mL of our final solution by dividing by 1,000:

$$1\,mL = \frac{125}{1,000}\ mg$$

STEP THREE

Now calculate the total amount for the volume required, i.e. multiply the amount for 1 mL by 4,000:

$$4,000\ mL = \frac{125}{1,000} \times 4,000 = 125 \times 4 = 500\ mg$$

STEP FOUR

Calculate the volume of the concentrated solution equivalent to 1 mg:

20,000 ppm means 20,000 g per 1,000,000 mL or 20,000 mg in 1,000 mL

$$1\,mg = \frac{1,000}{20,000}\ mL$$

STEP FIVE

To find out how much of the concentrated solution is needed, multiply the total number of milligrams in the final solution (Step 3 = 500 mg) by the volume for 1 mg of concentrated solution (Step 4), i.e.

$$500\ mg = \frac{1,000}{20,000} \times 500 = \frac{1,000}{40} = 25\ mL$$

Therefore 25 mL of the concentrated solution (20,000 ppm) is required.

Checking the calculated answer of 25 mL with our estimate of 25 mL means that we should be confident that our calculated answer is correct.

ANSWER: 25 mL of a 20,000 ppm (0.2% w/v) concentrated solution when made up to 4 litres (4,000 mL) will give a 125 ppm solution.

A formula can be used:

$$\frac{\text{Volume of stock}}{\text{solution (mL)}} = \frac{\text{Concentration of the final solution}}{\text{Concentration of the stock solution}} \times \frac{\text{Final volume}}{\text{needed (mL)}}$$

where:
Concentration of the final solution = 125 ppm
Concentration of the stock solution = 20,000 ppm
Final volume needed (mL) = 4,000 mL

Substitute the numbers into the formula:

$$\frac{125}{20,000} \times 4,000 = 25 \text{ mL}$$

ANSWER: 25 mL of a 20,000 ppm (0.2% w/v) concentrated solution when made up to 4 litres (4,000 mL) will give a 125 ppm solution.

PROBLEMS

Question 11   Adrenaline/epinephrine is sometimes combined with lidocaine when used as a local anaesthetic, usually as a 1 in 200,000 strength. How much adrenaline/epinephrine is there in a 20 mL vial?

Question 12   It is recommended that children should have fluoride supplements for their teeth if the fluoride content of drinking water is 0.7 ppm or less. How much is this when expressed as a concentration of micrograms per litre?

Answers can be found in Chapter 15.

DRUGS EXPRESSED IN UNITS

Doses of drugs that are derived from large biological molecules are expressed in units rather than weights. Such large molecules are difficult to purify and so rather than use a weight it is more accurate to use the biological activity of the drug which is expressed in units. Examples of such drugs are heparin and insulin.

The word 'units' should be written out in full, as the letter 'U' can be mistaken for a zero, or 'IU' (international units) can be mistaken for the number 10. These abbreviations can lead to dosage errors.

The calculation of doses and their translation into suitable dosage forms are similar to the calculations elsewhere in this chapter.

Heparin

Unfractionated heparin (UFH) is given subcutaneously or by continuous intravenous infusion. Infusions are usually given over 24 hours and the dose is adjusted according to laboratory results. However, low molecular weight heparin (LMWH) differs from unfractionated heparin (UFH) in its molecular size and weight, method of preparation and anticoagulant properties. The anticoagulant response to LMWH is highly correlated with body weight, allowing administration of a fixed dose, usually in terms of a patient's body weight.

Confusion can occur between units and volume; the following case report illustrates the point that care must be taken when prescribing and administering LMWHs.

BEWARE DOSING ERRORS WITH LOW MOLECULAR WEIGHT HEPARIN

Case report

A retired teacher was admitted to hospital with acute shortage of breath and was diagnosed as having a pulmonary embolus. She was prescribed subcutaneous tinzaparin, in a dose of 0.45 mL from a 20,000 unit per mL prefilled 0.5 mL syringe. Due to confusion over the intended dose, two 0.5 mL prefilled syringes or 20,000 units of tinzaparin were administered in error by the ward nursing staff on four consecutive days. As a result of this cumulative administration error the patient died due to a brain haemorrhage which, in the opinion of the pathologist, was due to the overdose of tinzaparin.

It was the prescriber's intention that the patient should receive 9,000 units of tinzaparin each day, but this information was not written on the prescription. The ward sister told a coroner's court hearing that the prescription was ambiguous. The dose was written as 0.45 mL and then 20,000 units, with the rest illegible. Due to this confusion the patient received an overdose and died.

From *Pharmacy in Practice* 2000; 10:260.

Insulin

The majority of patients now use an insulin device (such as a 'pen'), as they are convenient to use. However, the insulin syringe may still be used in the ward setting when the pen device is not available.

There are no calculations involved in the administration of insulin. Insulin comes in cartridges or vials containing 100 units/mL, and the doses prescribed are written in units. However, there is now an insulin that is available in two strengths – 100 units/mL and 200 units/mL – insulin degludec. Therefore, all you have to do is to dial or draw up the required dose using a pen device or an insulin syringe.

Insulin syringes are calibrated as 100 units in 1 mL and are available as 1 mL and 0.5 mL syringes.

So if the dose is 30 units, you simply draw up to the 30 unit mark on the syringe.

PART II: Performing calculations

The chapters in this section cover the type of drug calculations encountered in clinical situations on a daily basis:

- Simple dosage calculations
- More complex calculations, especially those encountered with
  - Paediatrics
  - Prescribing
- Infusion rate calculations

CHAPTERS IN THIS PART

7 DOSAGE CALCULATIONS

OBJECTIVES

At the end of this chapter, you should be familiar with the following:

- Calculation of the number of tablets or capsules required
- Drug dosages based on patient parameters (body weight or body surface area)
- Ways of expressing doses
- Calculation of dosages
- Displacement values or volumes
- Prescriber calculations

KEY POINTS

Calculating the number of tablets or capsules required

$$\text{number required} = \frac{\text{amount prescribed}}{\text{amount in each tablet or capsule}}$$

Dosages based on patient parameters

- Weight (dose/kg): dose × body weight (kg)
- Surface area (dose/m^2): dose × body surface area (m^2)

Ways of expressing doses

A dose can be described as a:

- single dose – sometimes referred to as a 'STAT' dose meaning 'at once' from the Latin *statum.*
- daily dose: e.g. atorvastatin 10 mg once daily.
- weekly dose: methotrexate, when used in rheumatoid arthritis.
- total daily dose given in three or four divided doses.

Calculating doses

- To be sure that your answer is correct, it is best to calculate from first principles (for example, using the one unit rule).
- If using a formula – make sure that the figures are entered correctly.
- Ensure that everything is in the same units.
- Always recheck your answer – if in any doubt, stop and get help.
- Ask yourself: Does my answer seem reasonable?

$$\frac{\text{amount you want}}{\text{amount you've got}} \times \text{volume it's in}$$

Displacement values or volumes

• Dry powder injections need to be reconstituted with a diluent before they are used. Sometimes the final volume of the injection will be greater than the volume of liquid that was added to the powder. This volume difference is called the injection's displacement value.

Volume to be added = Diluent volume − Displacement volume

INTRODUCTION

Dosage calculations are the basic everyday type of calculations you will be doing on the ward. They include calculating number of tablets or capsules required, divided doses, simple drug dosages, and dosages based on patient parameters, e.g. weight and body surface area.

It is important that you are able to do these calculations confidently, as mistakes may result in the patient receiving the wrong dose which may lead to serious consequences for the patient.

Hutton (2009) devised a five-step approach for dealing with drug calculations:

Step 1: Extract the relevant information from the prescription.
Step 2: Check if the available medicine is in the same units as the prescribed dose.
Step 3: For the dose prescribed, estimate whether you need more or less than the medicine on hand.
Step 4: Calculate the dose to be given.
Step 5: Check that your answer is around the estimated amount and is a sensible amount to be given by the prescribed route.

Don't forget to include the units for numbers as this will give you a 'sense of number' and enable you to put the answer into the correct clinical context.

After completing this chapter, you should not only be able to do the calculations, but you should also know how to decide whether your answer is reasonable.

CALCULATING THE NUMBER OF TABLETS OR CAPSULES REQUIRED

On the drug round, you will usually have available the strength of the tablets or capsules for the dose prescribed on a patient's drug chart (e.g. dose prescribed is furosemide 40 mg; tablets available are

furosemide 40 mg). However, there
may be instances when the strength
of the tablets or capsules available
may not match the dose prescribed
and you will have to calculate how
many tablets or capsules to give the
patient.

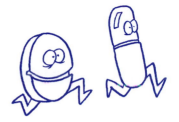

WORKED EXAMPLES

A patient is prescribed 75 micrograms of levothyroxine but the
strength of the tablets available is 25 micrograms. How many tablets
are required?

Before attempting the calculation, first estimate the answer.

First – check whether the dose prescribed and the medicine on
hand are in the same units; in this case, both have the same units and
so no conversion is needed.

Next, repeatedly add the strength for each tablet until you have
reached the dose prescribed:

25 micrograms – one

50 micrograms – two

75 micrograms – three

Although you have calculated the number of tablets needed, it is
always a good idea to do the calculation to check that you have the
right answer.

Now we can attempt the calculation.

This is a very simple calculation. The answer involves finding how
many 25s are in 75, or in other words 75 divided by 25 which equals:

$$\frac{75}{25} \text{ or } 3 = 3 \text{ tablets}$$

In most cases, it is a simple sum you can do in your head, but even so,
it is a drug calculation – so care must always be taken.

A patient is prescribed 2 g of flucloxacillin to be given orally but is available
in 500 mg capsules. How many capsules do you give now?

Before attempting the calculation, first estimate the answer.

Once again it is a simple calculation but it is slightly more complicated than our earlier example as the dose prescribed and the medicine on hand are in different units.

The first step is to convert everything to the same units. We could either convert the 500 mg into grams, or we could convert the 2 g into milligrams.

However, it is preferable to convert the grams to milligrams as this avoids decimal points.

Remember it is best not to work with decimal points – a decimal point in the wrong place can mean a 10-fold or even a 100-fold error.

To convert grams to milligrams – multiply by 1,000:

$$2 \text{ g} = 2 \times 1,000 = 2,000 \text{ mg}$$

Don't forget to estimate your answer – in this case, you can double the amount in each capsule until you have reached the dose prescribed.

500 mg – one

1,000 mg – two

2,000 mg – four

Although you have calculated the number of capsules needed, it is always a good idea to do the calculation to check that you have the right answer.

The calculation is now similar to our earlier example. The answer involves finding how many 500s are in 2,000 or in other words 2,000 divided by 500 which equals:

$$\frac{2000}{500} \text{ or } \frac{4}{1} = 4 \text{ capsules}$$

Once again, it is a simple sum you can do in your head, but it is a drug calculation – so care must always be taken.

A formula can be derived:

$$\text{Number required} = \frac{\text{amount prescribed}}{\text{amount in each tablet or capsule}}$$

If any calculation gives a dose of more than four tablets, double-check the calculation and confirm that the dose doesn't exceed the manufacturer's recommended maximum dose.

However, always try and give as few as possible – if the dose is 100 mg, give 2 × 50 mg rather than 4 × 25 mg.

For dosage calculations involving liquids and injections, see the section Calculating Drug Dosages.

Reference

Hutton M. Numeracy and drug calculations in practice. *Primary Health Care* 2009; 19(5): 40–45.

PROBLEMS

Question 1   Codeine 60 mg is prescribed. You have 15 mg and 30 mg tablets on-hand. Which tablets would you choose and how many would you give?

Question 2   Warfarin 2.5 mg is prescribed. You have 0.5 mg, 1 mg, 3 mg, and 5 mg tablets on hand. Which tablets would you choose and how many would you give?

Question 3   Alfacalcidol 1 microgram is prescribed. If you only have 250 nanograms capsules, how many would you give?

Answers can be found in Chapter 15.

DRUG DOSAGES BASED ON PATIENT PARAMETERS

Sometimes the dose required is calculated on a body weight basis (mg/kg) or in terms of a patient's surface area (mg/m^2). Using body surface area (BSA) estimates is more accurate than using body weight, since many physical phenomena are more closely related to the BSA. This particularly applies to cytotoxics and other drugs that require an accurate individual dose. To find the BSA for a patient, you will need to know that patient's height and weight. Then the BSA can be calculated, using a formula or nomograms (see Appendix 1).

However, for the majority of drugs, dosing on a weight basis is sufficient, particularly for children.

A caution about dosing by weight: For the majority of patients the actual (total) body weight (ABW or TBW) is the weight to be considered for dosing drugs. It is generally only when patients come within the definition of 'obese' (BMI >30) that significant effects on drug handling may be seen. In the case of obese patients, they may receive an artificially high dose. The reason for this is that fat tissue plays virtually no part in metabolism (including drug clearance) – using the ideal body weight (IBW) may be more appropriate.

WORKED EXAMPLES
Weight

The dose required is 3 mg/kg and the patient weighs 68 kg.

This means that for every kilogram (kg) of a patient's weight, you will need 3 mg of drug.

Before attempting the calculation, first estimate the answer.

In this case; you could round up the weight to 70 kg. This will give a dose of $3 \times 70 = 210$ mg. As the weight was rounded up, then the actual answer should be just below 210; a good guess would be 200 mg.

Now we can attempt the calculation.

In this example, the patient weighs 68 kg.

Therefore this patient will need 68 lots of 3 mg of drug, i.e. you simply multiply the dose by the patient's weight:

$$3 \text{ mg/kg} = 3 \times 68 = 204 \text{ mg}$$

Thus the patient will need a total dose of 204 mg.

Checking the calculated answer of 204 mg with our estimate of 200 mg means that we should be confident that our calculation is correct.

This can be summarized as:

$$\text{Total dose required} = \text{dose/kg} \times \text{patient's weight}$$

Surface area

Doses are calculated in the same way, substituting surface area for weight.

The dose required is 500 mg/m^2 and the patient's body surface area equals 1.89 m^2.

This means that for every square metre (m^2) of a patient's surface area, you will need 500 mg of drug. The dose is given in mg/m^2, so you multiply the dose by the patient's surface area.

Before attempting the calculation, first estimate the answer.

In this case, you can estimate by using a minimum and maximum (or a range). The BSA is 1.89 m^2 – this can be rounded down to 1.5 and rounded up to 2.

This will give a range of $500 \times 1.5 = 750$ and $500 \times 2 = 1,000$; 1.89 is toward the top of the range and a good guess would be 900 mg.

Now we can attempt the calculation.

In this example, the patient's body surface area is 1.89 m^2.

Therefore, this patient will need 1.89 lots of 500 mg of drug, i.e. you simply multiply the dose by the patient's body surface area (obtained from a formula or nomograms – see Appendix 1):

$$500 \text{ mg/m}^2 = 500 \times 1.89 = 945 \text{ mg}$$

Thus the patient will need a total dose of 945 mg.

Checking the calculated answer of 945 mg with our estimate of 900 mg means that we should be confident that our calculation is correct.

This can be summarized as:

$$\text{Total dose required} = \text{dose/m}^2 \times \text{body surface area}$$

PROBLEMS

Work out the following dosages:

Question 4   Dose = 1.5 mg/kg, patient's weight = 73 kg

Question 5   Dose = 60 mg/kg, patient's weight = 12 kg

Question 6   Dose = 50 mg/m^2, patient's surface area = 1.94 m^2

Question 7   Dose = 120 mg/m^2, patient's surface area = 1.55 m^2

Question 8   Dose = 400 mcg/kg, patient's weight = 54 kg

    i)   What is the total dose in micrograms?

    ii)   What is the total dose in mg?

Question 9   Dose = 5 mcg/kg/min, patient's weight = 65 kg

    i)   What is the dose in mcg/min? (You will meet this type of calculation with IV infusions.)

The following table will be needed to answer Questions 10 and 11.

LMWH	STRENGTH	PREPARATIONS AVAILABLE
Enoxaparin	• 150 mg/mL (15,000 units/mL) • Graduated in 0.02 mL (3 mg) increments	• 0.8 mL syringe (12,000 units, 120 mg) • 1 mL syringe (15,000 units, 150 mg)
Tinzaparin	• 20,000 units/mL • Graduated in 0.05 mL (1,000 units) increments	• 0.5 mL syringe (10,000 units) • 0.7 mL syringe (14,000 units) • 0.9 mL syringe (18,000 units)

Question 10   A patient has a deep vein thrombosis (DVT) and needs to be given tinzaparin at a dose of 175 units/kg. The patient weighs 74 kg. What dose does the patient need? Which syringe do you use and what volume do you give?

Question 11   A patient has a DVT and needs to be given enoxaparin at a dose of 1.5 mg/kg. The patient weighs 72 kg. What dose does the patient need? Which syringe do you use and what volume do you give?

Question 12   Using the Mosteller BSA formula (see Appendix 1):

$$m^2 = \sqrt{\frac{\text{height}(\text{cm}) \times \text{weight}(\text{kg})}{3600}}$$

Find out the BSA for a child weighing 20 kg and with a height of 108 cm. Calculate the answer to two decimal places.

Question 13   Using the Mosteller BSA formula (see Appendix 1):

$$m^2 = \sqrt{\frac{\text{height}(\text{cm}) \times \text{weight}(\text{kg})}{3600}}$$

Find out the BSA for a patient weighing 96 kg and with a height of 180 cm. Calculate the answer to two decimal places.

Answers can be found in Chapter 15.

WAYS OF EXPRESSING DOSES

A dose is the quantity or amount of a drug taken by, or administered to, a patient to achieve a therapeutic outcome.

A dose can be described as a **single** dose, a **daily** dose, a **daily divided** dose, a **weekly** dose, a **total** dose, etc. as described with examples below:

- Single dose: for example, premedication drugs. This is sometimes referred to as a 'STAT' dose meaning 'at once' from the Latin *statum*.
- Daily dose: for example, the BNF recommended dose of atorvastatin is 10 mg once daily
- Weekly dose: methotrexate, when used in rheumatoid arthritis
- Divided or total daily dose: the BNF for Children recommends for cefradine:
  By mouth
    Child 7–12 years
    12.5–25 mg/kg twice daily (total daily dose may alternatively be given in 3–4 divided doses)

In the above example, the dose can be given at the stated dose (twice daily) or as a total daily dose (TDD), given in divided doses (three or four times a day). This is particularly associated with paediatric doses. This is to allow flexibility in dosing – dosing on a weight basis may give a dose that cannot be given in two doses but can be given in three or four doses.

It is important that you can tell the difference between the TDD and individual doses. If not interpreted properly, then the patient is at risk of receiving the TDD as an individual dose, thus receiving three or four times the normal dose (with possible disastrous results).

CALCULATING DRUG DOSAGES

There are several ways of solving this type of calculation. It is best to learn one way and stick to it.

The easiest way is by proportion: what you do to one side of an equation, do the same to the other side. This is the one unit rule described in Chapter 1, and this method of calculation will be used here.

Also, when what you've got and what you want are in different units, you need to convert everything to the same units. When converting to the same units, it is best to convert to whole numbers to avoid decimal points as fewer mistakes are then made. If possible, it is a good idea to convert everything to the units of the answer.

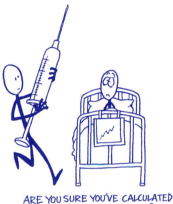

ARE YOU SURE YOU'VE CALCULATED THE DOSE CORRECTLY?

WORKED EXAMPLE

You need to give a patient 125 micrograms of digoxin orally. You have digoxin liquid 50 micrograms/mL supplied with a dropper pipette. How much do you need to draw up?

Before attempting the calculation, first estimate the answer.

Both the prescribed dose and the medicine on hand are in the same units, so no conversion is needed.

We have: 50 micrograms in 1 mL
So: 100 micrograms in 2 mL   (by doubling)
So: 25 micrograms in 0.5 mL   (by halving)
It follows: 125 micrograms in 2.5 mL   (by addition; 100 mcg + 25 mcg or 2 mL + 0.5 mL)

Now we can attempt the calculation.

STEP ONE

Write down what you have: 50 micrograms in 1 mL.

STEP TWO

Calculate how much **one** unit is of what you have, i.e.:

$$50 \text{ micrograms in 1 mL}$$

$$\text{microgram} = \frac{1}{50} \text{ mL}$$

This is the **one unit** rule.

STEP THREE

You need to know how much digoxin to draw up for 125 micrograms; therefore, multiply the amount from Step Two by 125:

$$125 \text{ micrograms} = \frac{1}{50} \times 125 = 2.5 \text{ mL}$$

ANSWER: You will need to draw up 2.5 mL of digoxin.

Checking the calculated answer of 2.5 mL with our estimate of 2.5 mL means that we should be confident that our calculation is correct.

From the above, a formula can be used to calculate drug dosages:

$$\frac{\text{amount you want}}{\text{amount you've got}} \times \text{volume it's in}$$

This formula should be familiar as this is the one universally taught for calculating doses. Remember, care must be taken when using any formula – ensure that numbers are entered and calculated correctly.

From the above example:

$$\text{amount you want} = 125 \text{ micrograms}$$

$$\text{amount you've got} = 50 \text{ micrograms}$$

$$\text{volume it's in} = 1 \text{ ml}$$

Substitute the numbers in the formula:

$$\frac{125}{50} \times 1 = 2.5 \text{ mL}$$

ANSWER: You will need to draw up 2.5 mL of digoxin.

You can apply this method to whatever type of calculation you want.

TIP BOX

There are several ways of solving these types of calculation. It is best to learn one way and stick to it.

The following case report illustrates the importance of ensuring that your calculations are right.

A PROBLEM WITH A DECIMAL POINT

Case report

A female baby, born seven weeks prematurely, died at 28 hours old when a junior doctor miscalculated a dose of intravenous morphine resulting in the administration of a 100-times overdose. The doctor is reported to have worked out the dose on a piece of paper and then checked it on a calculator, but the decimal point was inserted in the wrong place and 15 instead of 0.15 milligrams was prescribed. The dose was then prepared and handed to the senior registrar who administered it without double-checking the calculation, and despite treatment with naloxone, the baby died 55 minutes later.

From *Pharmacy in Practice* 1997; 7:368–369.

The following two case reports illustrate the importance of checking numbers before administration.

BE ALERT TO HIGH NUMBERS OF DOSE UNITS

Case one

A male patient was prescribed a stat dose of 2 g amiodarone for conversion of atrial fibrillation. Although it is still not known whether this dose was chosen deliberately or prescribed in error, there is evidence to support the use of a 2 g oral regimen. What concerned the reporting hospital was that the nurse administered 10 × 200 mg tablets to the patient without any reference or confirmation that this was indeed what was intended. This use of amiodarone is at present outside the product licence and would not have been described in any of the literature available on the ward.

The patient subsequently died but at the time of writing no causal effect from this high dose of amiodarone had been established.

Case two

A female patient aged approximately 65 was prescribed 2,500 units of dalteparin sodium subcutaneously once a day as part of the DVT prophylaxis protocol. The prescribed dose was misread and two nurses checking each other gave five prefilled syringes, i.e. 25,000 units, to the patient in error.

So much heparin was required that another patient's supply had to be used as well and the error came to light when the ward made a request to pharmacy for 25,000 unit doses of dalteparin. When the error was discovered the patient's coagulation status was checked immediately and she fortunately came to no harm.

Comment

It seems inconceivable that such high numbers of dose units could be administered to patients without the nurses involved at least querying that something might be wrong.

From *Pharmacy in Practice* 2001; 6:194.

PROBLEMS

Question 14 You need to give 1 g of erythromycin orally. You have erythromycin suspension 250 mg in 5 mL. How much of the suspension do you need to give?

Question 15 You need to give a patient 62.5 micrograms of digoxin orally. You have digoxin liquid containing 50 micrograms/mL. How much do you need to draw up?

Question 16 If Oramorph® concentrate 100 mg/5 mL is used to give a dose of 60 mg for breakthrough pain, what volume is required?

Question 17 You have pethidine injection 100 mg in 2 mL. The patient is prescribed 75 mg. How much do you draw up?

Question 18 You need to give ranitidine liquid at a dose of 2 mg/kg to a 9-year-old child weighing 23 kg. You have a 150 mg in 10 mL liquid. How much do you need to give for each dose?

Question 19 You need to give a dose of trimethoprim suspension to a child weighing 18.45 kg at a dose of 4 mg/kg. You have trimethoprim suspension 50 mg in 5 mL. What dose do you need to give and how much of the suspension do you need?

Question 20 Ciclosporin has been prescribed to treat a patient with severe rheumatoid arthritis. The oral dose is 2.5 mg/kg daily in two divided doses. The patient weighs 68 kg. Ciclosporin is available in 10 mg, 25 mg, 50 mg and 100 mg capsules. What dose is required and which strength of capsules would you need to give?

Question 21 You need to give aciclovir as an infusion at a dose of 5 mg/kg every 8 hours. The patient weighs 76 kg and aciclovir is available as 250 mg vials. How many vials do you need for each dose?

Question 22 A 50 kg woman is prescribed aminophylline as an infusion at a dose of 0.5 mg/kg/hour. Aminophylline injection comes as 250 mg in 10 mL ampoules. How much is required if the infusion is to run for 12 hours?

Question 23 You need to prepare an infusion of co-trimoxazole at a dose of 120 mg/kg/day in four divided doses for a patient weighing 78 kg. Co-trimoxazole is available as 5 mL ampoules at a strength of 96 mg/mL.

    i) What volume of co-trimoxazole do you need for each dose?

    ii) How many ampoules do you need for each dose?

    iii) How many ampoules do you need for 3 days (to cover a weekend)?

    iv) Before administration, co-trimoxazole must be diluted further: 1 ampoule diluted to 125 mL. In what volume should each dose be given? Round this up to the nearest commercially available bag size, i.e. 50 mL, 100 mL, 250 mL, 500 mL or 1 L.

Answers can be found in Chapter 15.

DISPLACEMENT VALUES OR VOLUMES

Dry powder injections need to be reconstituted with a diluent before they are used. Sometimes the final volume of the injection will be greater than the volume of liquid that was added to the powder. This volume difference is called the injection's displacement value.

What is displacement?

If you take ordinary salt and dissolve it in some water, the resultant solution will have a greater volume than before. The salt appears to 'displace' some water increasing the volume.

    Antibiotic suspensions are good examples to illustrate displacement.

    For example, to make up 100 mL of amoxicillin suspension, only 68 mL of water needs to be added. The amoxicillin powder must therefore displace 32 mL of water, i.e. 100 − 68 = 32 mL.

Is displacement important in medicine?

For most patients displacement of dry powder injections does not matter because the whole vial is administered. However it can be very important when you want to give a dose that is less than the total contents of the vial – a frequent occurrence for children and babies.

    The volume of the final solution must be considered when calculating the amount to withdraw from the vial. The total volume may be increased significantly and, if not taken into account, significant errors in dosage may occur, especially when small doses are involved as with babies.

For example:

Cefotaxime at a dose of 50 mg/kg, 12 hourly for a baby weighing 3.6 kg

Therefore dose required = 50 × 3.6 = 180 mg

Displacement volume for cefotaxime = 0.2 mL for a 500 mg vial

Therefore you need to add 1.8 mL (2 – 0.2) water for injection to give a final concentration of 500 mg in 2 mL. Thus:

$$180 \text{ mg} = \frac{2}{500} \times 180 = 0.72 \text{ mL}$$

If the displacement volume is not taken into account, then you will have:

500 mg in 2.2 mL (2 mL + 0.2 mL displacement volume)

You worked out earlier that the dose required is 180 mg and this is equal to 0.72 mL (assuming you have 500 mg in 2 mL). But actually 0.72 mL equals:

$$\frac{500}{2.2} \times 0.72 = 164 \text{ mg}$$

(The actual volume you have is 2.2 mL and *not* 2 mL.)

Thus if the displacement volume is not taken into account, then the amount drawn up is 164 mg and not 180 mg as expected.

Displacement values will depend on the medicine, the manufacturer and its strength. Information on a medicine's displacement value is usually stated in the relevant drug information sheets, in paediatric dosage books or can be obtained from your pharmacy department.

Calculating doses using displacement volumes is as follows:

volume to be added = diluent volume – displacement volume

For example, **benzylpenicillin**:

Dose required = 450 mg
Displacement volume = 0.4 mL per 600 mg vial
Diluent to be added = 5 mL
Volume to be added = 5 – 0.4 = 4.6 mL
Final concentration = 120 mg/mL
Volume required = 3.75 mL

PROBLEMS

Work out the following dosages, not forgetting to take into account displacement values if necessary.

Question 24   You need to give a 4-month-old child 350 mg ceftriaxone IV daily. You have a 1 g vial that needs to be reconstituted to 10 mL with Water for Injections. Displacement value = 0.8 mL for 1 g.

    i) Taking into account displacement volumes, what volume should you add to the vial?

    ii) How much do you need to draw up for each dose?

Question 25   You need to give cefotaxime IV to a 5-year-old child weighing 18 kg at a dose of 150 mg/kg/day in four divided doses. You have a 1 g vial that needs to be reconstituted to 4 mL with Water for Injections. Displacement value = 0.5 mL for 1 g.

    i) Taking into account displacement volumes, what volume should you add to the vial?

    ii) How much do you need to draw up for each dose?

Question 26   You need to give flucloxacillin IV to an 8-year-old child weighing 19.6 kg. The dose is 12.5 mg/kg four times a day. You have a 250 mg vial that needs to be reconstituted to 5 mL with Water for Injections. Displacement value = 0.2 mL for 250 mg.

    i) Taking into account displacement volumes, what volume should you add to the vial?

    ii) How much do you need to draw up for each dose?

Answers can be found in Chapter 15.

PRESCRIBER CALCULATIONS

The role of a nurse prescriber demands that there will be a greater number of drug calculations to be carried out and therefore accuracy in drug calculations is more important than ever (Axe 2001). In addition to the basic calculations for dosing, nurse prescribers need to be able to calculate the amount needed to complete the desired treatment course when writing a prescription.

Gregory (2002) cited in Hutton (2003) reminds us that 'a prescription can be viewed as a cheque on the NHS bank account. We should be as prudent as we would be in writing a cheque on our personal accounts'. In essence, prescribers need to be aware of what products are available and their costs so that the most cost-effective option can be chosen when several options are available.

References

Axe S. Numeracy and nurse prescribing: do the standards achieve their aim? *Nurse Education in Practice* 2011; 11(5): 285–287.

Hutton M. Calculations for new prescribers. *Nursing Standard* 2003; 17(25): 47–51.

WORKED EXAMPLE

You want to prescribe codeine linctus 10 mL QDS for 7 days for a cough. Codeine linctus (15 mg/5 mL) is available in 100 mL bottles. How much should you prescribe to ensure at least 7 days of treatment?

This is a straightforward calculation, so estimation is not really needed.

First, calculate how much is needed per day.

Dose = 10 mL QDS or 10 mL four times a day; dose per day equals:

$$10 \times 4 = 40 \text{ mL}$$

Next, calculate the amount for the treatment course (7 days):

$$40 \times 7 = 280 \text{ mL}$$

Each bottle is available as a 100 mL bottle, so the number needed equals:

$$\frac{280}{100} = 2.8 \text{ bottles}$$

Round up to the nearest 'bottle' to ensure a sufficient amount for the desired treatment course.

ANSWER: Prescribe three 100 mL bottles.

PROBLEMS

Question 27 As a prescriber, you need to write a prescription for codeine syrup (25 mg/5 mL) for a patient with swallowing difficulties. You want to prescribe a sufficient amount to give a dose of 30 mg four times a day for 2 weeks.

    i) How much is required for the required dose?

    ii) How much is required for a two-week supply?

Question 28 You want to prescribe a reducing dose of prednisolone. Starting at 20 mg daily for a week, then reducing by 5 mg every week to a dose of 5 mg daily for a week, then reducing by 1 mg every 2 days until zero milligrams is reached. How many 5 mg and 1 mg tablets do you need to prescribe?

Question 29   You want to prescribe an antacid to a patient at a dose of 10 mL at QDS for 28 days. Two brands are available:

Brand A costs £4.20 per 300 mL bottle and

Brand B costs £5.20 per 500 mL bottle.

What is the most cost-effective option?

For the following question you need to consult a current copy of the *British National Formulary* (either online or hard copy).

Question 30   As a prescriber, you want to write a prescription for an increasing regimen of gabapentin for an adult patient with neuropathic pain. How much is required for a 2-week supply?

Answers can be found in Chapter 15.

OBJECTIVES

At the end of this chapter you should be familiar with the following:

- Drip rate calculations (drops/min)
- Conversion of dosages to mL/hour
- Conversion of mL/hour back to a dose
- Calculating the length of time for IV infusions

KEY POINTS

Drip rate calculations (drops/min)

- In all drip rate calculations, you have to remember that you are simply converting a volume to drops (or vice versa) and hours to minutes.

$$\text{drops/min} = \frac{\text{drops/mL of the giving set} \times \text{volume of the infusion (mL)}}{\text{number of hours the infusion is to run} \times 60}$$

Giving sets

- The standard giving set (SGS) has a drip rate of *20 drops per mL* for clear fluids (i.e. sodium chloride, glucose) and *15 drops per mL* for blood.
- The micro-drop giving set or burette has a drip rate of *60 drops per mL*.

Conversion of dosages to mL/hour

- In this type of calculation, it is best to convert the dose required to a volume in millilitres.
- Doses are expressed as mcg/kg/min.

$$\text{mL/hour} = \frac{\text{volume to be infused} \times \text{dose} \times \text{wgt} \times 60}{\text{amount of drug} \times 1,000}$$

60 converts minutes to hours

1,000 converts mcg to mg

Note:

- If doses are expressed in terms of milligrams, then there is no need to divide by 1,000.
- If doses are expressed as a total dose, i.e. dose/min, there is no need to multiply by the patient's weight.

Conversion of mL/hour back to a dose

- Sometimes it may be necessary to convert *mL/hour* back to the dose: *mg/min* or *mcg/min* and *mg/kg/min* or *mcg/kg/min*.

$$\text{mcg/kg/min} = \frac{\text{rate (mL/hour)} \times \text{amount of drug} \times 1{,}000}{\text{weight (kg)} \times \text{volume (mL)} \times 60}$$

60 converts minutes to hours

1,000 converts mcg to mg

Note:

- If doses are expressed in terms of milligrams, then there is no need to multiply by 1,000.
- If doses are expressed as a total dose, i.e. dose/min, there is no need to divide by the patient's weight.

Calculating the length of time for IV infusions

- Sometimes it may be necessary to calculate the number of hours an infusion should run at a specified rate. Also, it is a good way of checking your calculated drip rate for an infusion.

Manually controlled infusions

$$\frac{\text{number of hours the}}{\text{infusion is to run}} = \frac{\text{volume of the infusion}}{\text{rate (drops/min)} \times 60} \times \text{drip rate of giving set}$$

Infusion or syringe pumps

$$\frac{\text{number of hours the}}{\text{infusion is to run}} = \frac{\text{volume of the infusion}}{\text{rate (mL/hour)}}$$

INTRODUCTION

With infusions, there are two types of infusion rate calculations to be considered, those involving **drops/min** and those involving **mL/hour**. The first (drops/min) is mainly encountered when infusions are given under gravity as with fluid replacement. The second (mL/hour) is encountered when infusions have to be given accurately or in small volumes using infusion or syringe pumps – particularly if drugs have to be given as infusions.

It is important to follow the manufacturer's guidelines for the length of time for an infusion to be administered. So calculations must be accurate to prevent complications from the medicines being administered too quickly. For example, if vancomycin is administered too quickly, the patient may experience 'red man syndrome' (RMS). RMS is characterized by flushing, erythema and pruritus, usually affecting the upper body, neck and face; in extreme cases, hypotension and angioedema may occur.

DRIP RATE CALCULATIONS (drops/min)

To set up a manually controlled infusion accurately, you need to be able to count the number of drops per minute. To do this, equate the volume to be infused in terms of drops. This in turn depends upon the giving or administration set being used.

Giving sets

There are two giving sets:

- The standard giving set (SGS) has a drip rate of *20 drops per mL* for clear fluids (i.e. sodium chloride, glucose) and *15 drops per mL* for blood.
- The micro-drop giving set or burette has a drip rate of *60 drops per mL*.

The drip rate of the giving set is always written on the wrapper if you are not sure.

Before attempting any calculation, it is important to decide which giving set is appropriate.

In all drip rate calculations, remember that you are simply converting a volume to drops (or vice versa) and hours to minutes.

WORKED EXAMPLE

One litre of sodium chloride 0.9% is to be given over 8 hours. What drip rate is required using an SGS, 20 drops/mL?

Before attempting the calculation, first estimate the required drip rate.

$$1 \text{ litre} = 1,000 \text{ mL and}$$
$$8 \text{ hours} = 480 \text{ min (round up the time to 500 min)}$$

Convert the infusion to a number of drops:

$$1,000 \times 20 = 20,000 \text{ drops}$$

Therefore, drops per minute would equal

$$\frac{20,000}{500} = \frac{200}{5} = 40 \text{ drops/min}$$

As the length of time for the infusion was rounded up, then the actual drip rate will be slightly higher.

Now we can attempt the calculation.

STEP ONE

First convert the volume to a number of drops. To do this, multiply the volume of the infusion (in mL) by the number of drops per mL for the giving set, i.e.

$$1 \text{ litre} = 1{,}000 \text{ mL}$$

so it will be:

$$1{,}000 \times 20 = 20{,}000 \text{ drops}$$

Thus for the giving set being used, you have just calculated the number of drops to be infused.

STEP TWO

Next convert hours to minutes by multiplying the number of hours over which the infusion is to be given by 60 (60 minutes = 1 hour).

$$8 \text{ hours} = 8 \times 60 = 480 \text{ minutes}$$

Now everything has been converted in terms of drops and minutes, i.e. what you want for your final answer.

If the infusion is being given over a period of minutes, then obviously there is no need to convert from hours to minutes.

STEP THREE

Write down what you have just calculated, i.e. the total number of drops to be given over how many minutes:

$$20{,}000 \text{ drops to be given over } 480 \text{ minutes}$$

$$(20{,}000 \text{ drops} = 480 \text{ min})$$

STEP FOUR

Calculate the number of drops per minute by dividing the number of drops by the number of minutes, i.e.

$$20{,}000 \text{ drops over } 480 \text{ minutes}$$

$$\frac{20{,}000}{480} = 41.67 \text{ drops/min}$$

Since it is impossible to have part of a drop, round up or down to the nearest whole number:

$$41.67 = 42 \text{ drops/min}$$

ANSWER: To give a litre (1,000 mL) of sodium chloride 0.9% ('normal saline') over 8 hours, the rate will have to be 42 drops/min using an SGS (20 drops/mL).

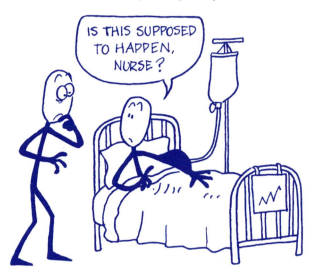

A formula can be used:

$$\text{drops/min} = \frac{\text{drops/mL of the giving set} \times \text{volume of the infusion (mL)}}{\text{number of hours the infusion is to run} \times 60}$$

where in this case:

Drops/mL of the giving set = 20 drops/mL (SGS)

Volume of the infusion (in mL) = 1,000 mL

Number of hours the infusion is to run = 8 hours

60 = number of minutes in an hour (converts hours to minutes)

Substitute the numbers in the formula:

$$\frac{20 \times 1,000}{8 \times 60} = 41.67 \text{ drops/min (42 drops/min, approx.)}$$

ANSWER: To give a litre (1,000 mL) of sodium chloride 0.9% ('normal saline') over 8 hours, the rate will have to be 42 drops/min using an SGS (20 drops/mL).

Note: If the rate is given in terms of mL/hour, then the drip rate can be easily calculated by dividing by three. For example, in the above example, the rate would be 125 mL/hour. Convert hours to minutes making the rate 125 mL/60 min; so the rate per minute would be:

$$\frac{125}{60}\, mL/min$$

Convert the volume to drops by multiplying by 20 (20 drops = 1 mL):

$$\frac{125}{60} \times 20 = \frac{125}{3} = drops/min$$

So $\frac{125}{3}$ = 41.67 drops/min.

PROBLEMS

Work out the drip rates for the following:

Question 1   500 mL of sodium chloride 0.9% over 6 hours

Question 2   1 litre of glucose 4% and sodium chloride 0.18% over 12 hours

Question 3   1 unit of blood (500 mL) over 6 hours

Answers can be found in Chapter 15.

CONVERSION OF DOSAGES TO mL/hour

Dosages can be expressed in various ways: *mg/min* or *mcg/min* and *mg/kg/min* or *mcg/kg/min*; it may be necessary to convert to *mL/hour* (when using infusion pumps). Ensure that you take into account the relevant conversion factors – should the answer be in terms of mL/min or mL/hour?

The following example shows the various steps in this type of calculation, and this can be adapted to any dosage to infusion rate calculation.

WORKED EXAMPLES

You have an infusion of dopamine 800 mg in 500 mL. The dose required is 2 mcg/kg/min for a patient weighing 68 kg. What is the rate in mL/hour?

Before attempting the calculation, first estimate the required infusion rate. Round up the patient's weight to 70 kg

Dose required = 70 × 2 = 140 mcg/min

Find the amount per hour (by multiplying by 60):

$$140 \times 60 = 8,400 \text{ mcg/hour}$$

As the dose and medicine on hand are in different units – convert to the same units (convert micrograms to milligrams by dividing by 1,000).

$$8,400 \text{ mcg} = 8,400/1,000 = 8.4 \text{ mg}$$

We have 800 mg – 500 mL, so

400 mg	–	250 mL (by halving)
200 mg	–	125 mL (by halving)
100 mg	–	62.5 mL (by halving)
10 mg	–	6.25 mL (dividing by 10)
1 mg	–	0.625 mL (dividing by 10)
8 mg	–	5 mL (multiplying by 8)
0.1 mg	–	0.0625 mL (dividing by 10)
0.4 mg	–	0.25 mL (multiplying by 4)

It follows 8.4 mg – 5.25 mL (by addition; 8 mg + 0.4 mg or 5 mL + 0.25 mL).

As the weight has been rounded up, then the actual answer should be less than the estimated answer – around 5.2 mL/hour would be a good guess.

Now we can attempt the calculation.

STEP ONE

When answering this type of calculation, you need to convert the dose required to a volume in millilitres and minutes to hours.

STEP TWO

First calculate the dose required:

$$\text{dose required} = \text{patient's weight} \times \text{dose prescribed}$$
$$= 68 \times 2 = 136 \text{ mcg/min}$$

If the dose is given as a total dose and not on a weight basis, then miss out this step.

STEP THREE

The dose is 136 mcg/min. The final answer is in terms of hours, so multiply by 60 to convert minutes into hours:

$$\text{dose} = 136 \text{ mcg/min} = 136 \times 60 = 8,160 \text{ mcg/hour}$$

As the dose and drug are in different units – convert to the same units (convert micrograms to milligrams).

Convert mcg to mg by dividing by 1,000:

$$\frac{8,160}{1,000} = 8.16 \text{ mg/hour}$$

STEP FOUR

The next step is to calculate the volume for the dose required.

Calculate the volume for 1 mg of drug:

You have: 800 mg in 500 mL

$$1 \text{ mg} = \frac{500}{800} = 0.625 \text{ mL}$$

STEP FIVE

Thus for the dose of 8.16 mg, the volume is equal to:

$$8.16 \text{ mg} = 0.625 \times 8.16 = 5.1 \text{ mL/hour}$$

Either round up or down to a whole number or calculate to one or two decimal places depending upon the type of pump being used.

Checking the calculated answer of 5.1 mL/hour with our estimate of 5.2 mL/hour means that we should be confident that our calculated answer is correct.

ANSWER: The rate required = 5.1 mL/hour.

A formula can be derived:

$$\text{mL/hour} = \frac{\text{volume to be infused} \times \text{dose} \times \text{wgt} \times 60}{\text{amount of drug} \times 1,000}$$

In this case:

Total volume to be infused = 500 mL

Total amount of drug (mg) = 800 mg

Dose = 2 mcg/kg/min

Patient's weight (wgt) = 68 kg

60 converts minutes to hours

1,000 converts mcg to mg

Substitute the numbers in the formula:

$$\frac{500 \times 2 \times 68 \times 60}{800 \times 1,000} = 5.1 \text{ mL/hour}$$

ANSWER: The rate required = 5.1 mL/hour.

If the dose is given as a total dose and not on a weight basis, then the patient's weight is not needed.

$$mL/hour = \frac{\text{volume to be infused} \times \text{dose} \times 60}{\text{amount of drug} \times 1{,}000}$$

Note:

- If doses are expressed in terms of milligrams, then there is no need to divide by 1,000.
- If doses are expressed as a total dose, i.e. dose/min, there is no need to multiply by the patient's weight.

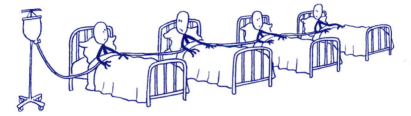

I KNOW THEY'RE SUPPOSED TO CUT COSTS,
BUT THIS IS RIDICULOUS !

Following on from this, instead of maintaining a single dose, it may be necessary to titrate the dose according to response. For dopamine, the dose can range from 2 to 5 mcg/kg/min, so it may be necessary to change the rate of an infusion partway through the administration.

In this situation, calculate the rate for a 'unit' dose, whether it's 1 mcg, 0.1 mcg or 0.01 mcg, and use this for multiples of dose.

In the above example, we would calculate the rate for 1 mcg/kg/min and adjust the rate for subsequent increments in dose if necessary.

Before attempting the calculation, first estimate the answer.

Round up the weight to 70 kg.

So the dose = 1 mcg/min × 70 kg = 70 mcg/min.

Multiply by 60 to convert to hours.

$$70 \times 60 = 4{,}200 \text{ mcg/hour}$$

As the dose and medicine on hand are in different units, convert to the same units (convert micrograms to milligrams by dividing by 1,000).

$$\frac{4{,}200}{1{,}000} = 4.2 \text{ mg/hour}$$

We have 800 mg – 500 mL, so

400 mg	–	250 mL (by halving)
200 mg	–	125 mL (by halving)
100 mg	–	62.5 mL (by halving)
10 mg	–	6.25 mL (dividing by 10)
1 mg	–	0.625 mL (dividing by 10)
4 mg	–	2.5 mL (multiplying by 4)
0.1 mg	–	0.0625 mL (dividing by 10)
0.2 mg	–	0.125 mL (multiplying by 2)

It follows 4.2 mg – 2.625 mL (by addition; 4 mg + 0.2 mg or 2.5 mL + 0.125 mL).

As the weight has been rounded up, then the actual answer should be less than the estimated answer – around 2.5 mL/hour would be a good guess.

Now we can attempt the calculation.

STEP ONE

First calculate the dose required for 1 mcg/kg/min for this patient:

dose required = patient's weight × 1 = 68 mcg/min

If the dose is given as a total dose and not on a weight basis, then miss out this step.

STEP TWO

The dose is 68 mcg/min. The final answer is in terms of hours, so multiply by 60 to convert minutes into hours:

dose = 68 mcg/min = 68 × 60 = 4,080 mcg/hour

As the dose and drug are in different units, convert to the same units (convert micrograms to milligrams).

Convert mcg to mg by dividing by 1,000:

$$\frac{4,080}{1,000} = 4.08 \text{ mg/hour}$$

STEP THREE

The next step is to calculate the volume for the dose required.
Calculate the volume for 1 mg of drug:
You have: 800 mg in 500 mL.

$$1 \text{ mg} = \frac{500}{800} = 0.625 \text{ mL}$$

STEP FOUR

Thus for the dose of 4.08 mg, the volume is equal to:

$$4.08 \text{ mg} = 0.625 \times 4.08 = 2.55 \text{ mL/hour}$$

Either round up or down to a whole number or calculate to one or two decimal places depending upon the type of pump being used.

Checking the calculated answer of 2.55 mL/hour with our estimate of 2.5 mL/hour means that we should be confident that our calculated answer is correct.

STEP FIVE

The next step is to calculate the rate for each dose required:

$$1 \text{ mcg/kg/min} = 2.55 \text{ mL/hour}$$
$$2 \text{ mcg/kg/min} = 5.1 \text{ mL/hour} \quad (2 \times 2.55)$$
$$3 \text{ mcg/kg/min} = 7.65 \text{ mL/hour} \quad (3 \times 2.55)$$
$$4 \text{ mcg/kg/min} = 10.2 \text{ mL/hour} \quad (4 \times 2.55)$$
$$5 \text{ mcg/kg/min} = 12.75 \text{ mL/hour} \quad (5 \times 2.55)$$

We can use the same formula:

$$\text{mL/hour} = \frac{\text{volume to be infused} \times \text{dose} \times \text{wgt} \times 60}{\text{amount of drug} \times 1{,}000}$$

In this case:

$$\text{Total volume to be infused} = 500 \text{ mL}$$
$$\text{Total amount of drug (mg)} = 800 \text{ mg}$$
$$\text{Unit dose} = 1 \text{ mcg/kg/min}$$
$$\text{Patient's weight (wgt)} = 68 \text{ kg}$$
$$60 \text{ converts minutes to hours}$$
$$1{,}000 \text{ converts mcg to mg}$$

Substitute the numbers in the formula:

$$\frac{500 \times 1 \times 68 \times 60}{800 \times 1{,}000} = 2.55 \text{ mL/hour}$$

The rate required for a unit dose = 2.55 mL/hour – from this, we can calculate the rates from 1 mcg/kg/min to 5 mcg/kg/min.

TABLE OF INFUSION RATES (ML/HOUR)

Time Vol	MINUTES					HOURS										
	10	15	20	30	40	1	2	3	4	6	8	10	12	16	18	24
10 mL	60	40	30	20												
20 mL	120	80	60	40												
30 mL				60												
40 mL				80	60	40										
50 mL				100	75	50										
60 mL				120	90	60										
80 mL				160	120	80										
100 mL				200	150	100	50	33	25	17						
125 mL				250	188	125	63	42	31	21						
150 mL				300	225	150	75	50	38	25						
200 mL				400	300	200	100	67	50	33	25	20	17	13	11	8
250 mL							125	83	63	42	31	25	21	16	14	10
500 mL									125	83	63	50	42	31	28	21
1,000 mL									250	167	125	100	83	63	56	42

Note: Rates given in the table have been rounded up or down to give whole numbers.

How to use the table

If you need to give a 250 mL infusion over 8 hours, then to find the infusion rate (mL/hour) go down the left hand (Vol) column until you reach 250 mL; then go along the top (Time) line until you reach 8 (for 8 hours). Then read off the corresponding infusion rate (mL/hour), in this case it equals 31 mL/hour.

PROBLEMS

Question 4 You have a 500 mL infusion containing 50 mg glyceryl trinitrate. A dose of 10 mcg/min is required. What is the rate in mL/hour?

Question 5 You are asked to give 500 mL of lidocaine 0.2% in glucose at a rate of 2 mg/min. What is the rate in mL/hour?

Question 6 A patient with chronic obstructive pulmonary disease (COPD) is to have a continuous infusion of aminophylline. The patient weighs 63 kg and the dose to be given is 0.5 mg/kg/hour over 12 hours. Aminophylline injection comes as 250 mg in 10 mL ampoules and should be given in a 500 mL infusion bag.

  a. What dose and volume of aminophylline are required?

  b. What is the rate in mL/hour?

Question 7 You need to give aciclovir as an infusion at a dose of 5 mg/kg every 8 hours. The patient weighs 86 kg and aciclovir is available as 500 mg vials. Each vial needs to be reconstituted with 20 mL water for injection and diluted further to 100 mL. The infusion should be given over 60 minutes.

  a. What dose and volume of aciclovir are required for one dose?

  b. What is the rate in mL/hour for each dose?

Question 8 Glyceryl trinitrate is to be given at a starting rate of 150 mcg/min. You have an infusion of 50 mg in 50 mL glucose 5%. What is the rate in mL/hour?

Question 9 A patient with methicillin-resistant *Staphylococcus aureus* (MRSA) is prescribed IV vancomycin 1 g every 24 hours. After reconstitution a 500 mg vial of vancomycin should be diluted with infusion fluid to 5 mg/mL.

  a. What is the minimum volume (mL) of infusion fluid that 1 g vancomycin can be administered in? (Round this to the nearest commercially available bag size, e.g. 50 mL, 100 mL, 250 mL, 500 mL or 1,000 mL.)

  b. The rate of administration should not exceed 10 mg/min. Over how many minutes should the infusion be given?

  c. What is the rate in mL/hour?

Question 10 You are asked to give an infusion of dobutamine to a patient weighing 73 kg at a dose of 5 mcg/kg/min. You have an infusion of 500 mL sodium chloride 0.9% containing one 250 mg of dobutamine.

    a. What is the dose required (mcg/min)?

    b. What is the concentration (mcg/mL) of dobutamine?

    c. What is the rate in mL/hour?

Question 11 You are asked to give an infusion of isosorbide dinitrate 50 mg in 500 mL of glucose 5% at a rate of 2 mg/hour.

    a. What is the rate in mL/hour? The rate is then changed to 5 mg/hour.

    b. What is the new rate in mL/hour?

Question 12 You have an infusion of dopamine 800 mg in 500 mL. The initial dose required is 2 mcg/kg/min and increases in increments of 1 mcg to a maximum of 10 mcg/kg/min. Patient's weight is 80 kg. What is the rate in mL/hour (one decimal place) for each incremental dose?

Question 13 You have an infusion of dobutamine 250 mg in 50 mL. The initial dose required is 2.5 mcg/kg/min and increases in increments of 2.5 mcg to a maximum of 10 mcg/kg/min. Patient's weight is 75 kg. What is the rate in mL/hour (one decimal place) for each incremental dose?

Answers can be found in Chapter 15.

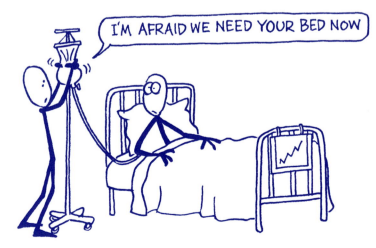

INCREASING THE INFUSION RATE

CONVERSION OF mL/hour BACK TO A DOSE

Sometimes it may be necessary to convert *mL/hour* back to the dose: *mg/min* or *mcg/min* and *mg/kg/min* or *mcg/kg/min*.

It is a good idea to regularly check that the infusion pump is set correctly – particularly in critical areas.

WORKED EXAMPLE
An infusion pump containing 250 mg dobutamine in 50 mL is running at a rate of 3.5 mL/hour. You want to convert back to mcg/kg/min to check that the pump is set correctly.

(Patient's weight = 73 kg and the prescribed dose is 4 mcg/kg/min.) Before attempting the calculation, first estimate the original dose. Don't forget, this is only an estimate – it will only detect large discrepancies, not small ones such as less than 0.5 mL.

The current rate is 3.5 mL/hour.

Next, we need to convert the volume to an amount.

We have 50 mL – 250 mg, so

$$5 \text{ mL} \quad - \quad 25 \text{ mg (dividing by 10)}$$
$$1 \text{ mL} \quad - \quad 5 \text{ mg (dividing by 5)}$$
$$0.5 \text{ mL} \quad - \quad 2.5 \text{ mg (dividing by 10)}$$
$$3 \text{ mL} \quad - \quad 15 \text{ mg (multiplying by 10)}$$

It follows: 3.5 mL – 17.5 mg (by addition; 3 mL + 0.5 mL or 25 mg + 2.5 mg).

The rate can be rewritten as 17.5 mg/hour.

The dose prescribed and the rate have different units, so a conversion is needed. Convert milligrams to micrograms – multiply by 1,000:

$$17.5 \times 1,000 = 17,500 \text{ mcg/hour}$$

Next convert to an amount per minute. For ease of calculation, round up the dose to 18,000 mcg/hour.

We have 18,000 mcg – 60 min, so

$$9,000 \text{ mcg} - 30 \text{ min (dividing by 2)}$$
$$3,000 \text{ mcg} - 10 \text{ min (dividing by 3)}$$

It follows: 300 mcg – 1 min (dividing by 10).

To calculate the dose, the weight needs to be taken into account; weight = 73 kg – round up to 75 kg. To find the dose, divide by the weight:

$$\frac{300}{75} = \frac{60}{15} = \frac{12}{3} = 4 \text{ mcg/kg/min}$$

As the rate and weight have been rounded up, the actual dose will be slightly less – but it will be rounded up, so 4 mcg/kg/min remains a good guess.

It has been estimated that the dose is correct and no adjustment is necessary.

Now we can attempt the calculation.

STEP ONE

In this type of calculation, convert the volume being given to the amount of drug, and then work out the amount of drug being given per minute or even per kilogram of the patient's weight.

STEP TWO

You have 250 mg of dobutamine in 50 mL.

Now it is necessary to work out the amount in 1 mL:

$$250 \text{ mg in } 50 \text{ mL}$$

$$1 \text{ mL} = \frac{250}{50} \text{ mg} = 5 \text{ mg} \qquad \text{(using the ONE unit rule)}$$

STEP THREE

The rate at which the pump is running is 3.5 mL/hour. You have just worked out the amount in 1 mL (Step two), therefore for 3.5 mL:

$$3.5 \text{ mL/hour} = 5 \times 3.5 = 17.5 \text{ mg/hour}$$

So the rate (mL/hour) has been converted to the amount of drug being given over an hour.

STEP FOUR

To make the figures easier to deal with, convert milligrams to micrograms by multiplying by 1,000:

$$17.5 \times 1,000 = 17,500 \text{ mcg/hour}$$

STEP FIVE

Now calculate the rate per minute by dividing by 60 (converts hours to minutes).

$$\frac{17,500}{60} = 291.67 \text{ mcg/min}$$

STEP SIX

The final step in the calculation is to work out the rate according to the patient's weight (73 kg). If the dose is not given in terms of the patient's weight, then miss out this final step.

$$\frac{291.67}{73} = 3.99 \text{ mcg/kg/min}$$

This can be rounded up to 4 mcg/kg/min.

Checking the calculated answer of 4 mcg/kg/min with our estimate of 4 mcg/kg/min means that we should be confident that our calculated answer is correct.

Now check your answer against the dose written on the drug chart to see if the pump is delivering the correct dose. If your answer does not match the dose written on the drug chart, then recheck your calculation. If the answer is still the same, then inform the doctor and, if necessary, calculate the correct rate.

ANSWER: The dose is correct. No adjustment is necessary.

A formula can be devised:

$$\text{mcg/kg/min} = \frac{\text{rate (mL/hour)} \times \text{amount of drug} \times 1,000}{\text{weight (kg)} \times \text{volume (mL)} \times 60}$$

where in this case:

$$\text{Rate} = 3.5 \text{ mL/hour}$$
$$\text{Amount of drug (mg)} = 250 \text{ mg}$$
$$\text{Weight (kg)} = 73 \text{ kg}$$
$$\text{Volume (mL)} = 50 \text{ mL}$$
$$60 \text{ converts minutes to hours}$$
$$1,000 \text{ converts mg to mcg}$$

Substitute the numbers in the formula:

$$\frac{3.5 \times 250 \times 1,000}{70 \times 50 \times 60} = 3.99 \text{ mcg/kg/min}$$

This can be rounded up to 4 mcg/kg/min.

ANSWER: The dose is correct. No adjustment is necessary.

If the dose is given as a total dose and not on a weight basis, then the patient's weight is not needed.

$$\text{mcg/min} = \frac{\text{rate (mL/hour)} \times \text{amount of drug} \times 1,000}{\text{volume (mL)} \times 60}$$

Note: If the dose is in terms of milligrams, then there is no need to multiply by 1,000 (i.e. delete from the formula).

PROBLEMS

Convert the following infusion pump rates to a mcg/kg/min dose.

Question 14   You have dopamine 200 mg in 50 mL and the rate at which the pump is running = 4 mL/hour. The prescribed dose is 3 mcg/kg/min.

What dose is the pump delivering?

(Patient's weight = 89 kg)

If the dose is wrong, at which rate should the pump be set?

Question 15   You have dobutamine 250 mg in 50 mL, and the rate at which the pump is running = 5.4 mL/hour. The prescribed dose is 6 mcg/kg/min.

What dose is the pump delivering?

(Patient's weight = 64 kg)

If the dose is wrong, at which rate should the pump be set?

Question 16   You have dopexamine 50 mg in 50 mL, and the rate at which the pump is running = 28 mL/hour. The prescribed dose is 6 mcg/kg/min.

What dose is the pump delivering?

(Patient's weight = 78 kg)

If the dose is wrong, at which rate should the pump be set?

Answers can be found in Chapter 15.

CALCULATING THE LENGTH OF TIME FOR IV INFUSIONS

It may sometimes be necessary to calculate the number of hours an infusion should run at a specified rate. This is also a good way of checking your calculated drip rate or pump rate for an infusion.

For example: You are asked to give a litre of 5% glucose over 8 hours.

You have calculated that the drip rate should be 42/drops/min (using an SGS: 20 drops/mL) or 125 mL/hour for a pump.

To check your answer, you can calculate how long the infusion should take at the calculated rate. If your answers do not correspond (the answer should be 8 hours), then you have made an error and should recheck your calculation.

Alternatively, you can use this type of calculation to check the rate of an infusion already running.

For example: If an infusion is supposed to run over 6 hours, and the infusion is nearly finished after 4 hours, you can check the rate by calculating how long the infusion should take using that drip rate or the rate set on the pump. If the calculated answer is less than 6 hours, then the original rate was wrong and the doctor should be informed, if necessary.

WORKED EXAMPLE
Manually controlled infusions

The doctor prescribes 1 litre of 5% glucose to be given over 8 hours. The drip rate for the infusion is calculated to be 42 drops/min. You wish to check the drip rate. How many hours is the infusion going to run? (SGS = 20 drops/mL)

Before attempting the calculation, first estimate the length of time for the infusion. In this case, convert drops to a volume and minutes to hours.

To make calculations easier, round down the drip rate to 40 drops/min.

We know that 20 drops equals to 1 mL; so 40 drops would equal to 2 mL.

Next, calculate the time taken to administer 1,000 mL (or 1 litre).

We have: 2 mL – 1 min
So: 200 mL – 100 min   (multiplying by 100)
It follows: 1,000 mL – 500 min   (multiplying by 5)
Finally, convert minutes to hours by dividing by 60:

$$\frac{500}{60} = \frac{50}{6} = \frac{25}{3} = 8.33 \text{ hours}$$

As the rate has been rounded down, the actual dose will be slightly less – around 8 hours would be a good guess.

Now we can attempt the calculation.

STEP ONE

In this calculation, you first convert the volume being infused to drops, then calculate how long it will take at the specified rate.

STEP TWO

First, convert the volume to drops by multiplying the volume of the infusion (in mL) by the number of drops/mL for the giving set.

volume of infusion = 1 litre = 1,000 mL, so it will be:

$1,000 \times 20 = 20,000$ drops

STEP THREE

From the rate, calculate how many minutes it will take for 1 drop, i.e.

$$42 \text{ drops per minute}$$

$$1 \text{ drop} = \frac{1}{42} \text{ min}$$

STEP FOUR

Calculate how many minutes it will take to infuse the total number of drops:

$$1 \text{ drop} = \frac{1}{42} \text{ min}$$

$$20,000 \text{ drops} = \frac{1}{42} \times 20,000 = 476 \text{ min}$$

STEP FIVE

Convert minutes to hours by dividing by 60:

$$476 \text{ min} = \frac{476}{60} = 7.93 \text{ hours}$$

How much is 0.93 of an hour?
Multiply by 60 to convert part of an hour back to minutes:

$$0.93 \times 60 = 55.8 \text{ min} = 56 \text{ min (approx.)}$$

Putting the two together will give an answer of approximately 8 hours (7 hours and 56 minutes).

Checking the calculated answer of 8 hours with our estimate of 8 hours means that we should be confident that our calculated answer is correct.

ANSWER: 1 litre of glucose 5% at a rate of 42 drops/min will take approximately 8 hours to run (7 hours and 56 min).

A formula can be used:

$$\text{number of hours the infusion is to run} =$$

$$\frac{\text{volume of the infusion}}{\text{rate (drops/min)} \times 60} \times \text{drip rate of giving set}$$

where in this case:

$$\text{Volume of the infusion} = 1,000 \text{ mL}$$
$$\text{Rate (drops/min)} = 42 \text{ drops/min}$$
$$\text{Drip rate of giving set} = 20 \text{ drops/mL}$$
$$60 \text{ converts minutes to hours}$$

Substitute the numbers in the formula:

$$\frac{1,000 \times 20}{42 \times 60} = 7.94 \text{ hours}$$

Convert 0.94 hours to minutes: = 56 min (approx.)

ANSWER: 1 litre of glucose 5% at a rate of 42 drops/min will take approximately 8 hours to run (7 hours 56 min).

WORKED EXAMPLE

Infusion or syringe pumps

The doctor prescribes 1 litre of 5% glucose to be given over 8 hours. The rate for the infusion is calculated to be 125 mL/hour. You wish to check the rate. How many hours is the infusion going to run?

Before attempting the calculation, first estimate the length of time for the infusion. The rate is 125 mL/hour, so:

calculated rate = 125 mL – 1 hour

So: 250 mL – 2 hours (by doubling)

So: 500 mL – 4 hours (by doubling)

It follows: 1,000 mL – 8 hours (by doubling)

Although we have calculated the length of time for the infusion, it is always a good idea to do the calculation to check that you have the right answer.

Now we can attempt the calculation.

This is a simple calculation. Divide the total volume (in mL) by the rate to give the time over which the infusion is to run.

calculated rate = 125 mL/hour

volume = 1,000 mL   (1 litre = 1,000 mL)

$$\frac{1,000}{125} = 8 \text{ hours}$$

Checking the calculated answer of 8 hours with our estimate of 8 hours means that we should be confident that our calculated answer is correct.

ANSWER: 1 litre of glucose 5% at a rate of 125 mL/hour will take 8 hours to run.

A simple formula can be used:

$$\text{number of hours the infusion is to run} = \frac{\text{volume of the infusion}}{\text{rate (mL/hour)}}$$

where in this case:

Volume of the infusion = 1,000 mL

Rate (mL/hour) = 125 mL/hour

Substitute the numbers in the formula:

$$\frac{1,000}{125} = 8 \text{ hours}$$

ANSWER: 1 litre of glucose 5% at a rate of 125 mL/hour will take 8 hours to run.

PROBLEMS

Question 17   A 500 mL infusion of sodium chloride 0.9% is being given over 4 hours. The rate at which the infusion is being run is 42 drops/min. How long will the infusion run at the specified rate? (SGS)

Question 18   A 1 L infusion of sodium chloride 0.9% is being given over 12 hours. The rate at which the infusion is being run is 83 mL/hour. How long will the infusion run at the specified rate?

Answers can be found in Chapter 15.

PART III: Administering medicines

This section covers the practical aspects of administration of medicines:

- How the body handles and respond to drugs
- Common routes of administration
- Specific groups of patients
  - Children
  - The elderly
- Sources and interpretation of drug information

CHAPTERS IN THIS PART

9 INTRAVENOUS THERAPY AND INFUSION DEVICES

OBJECTIVES

At the end of this chapter you should be familiar with the following:

- IV infusion therapy
  - Fluid balance in man
  - Infusion fluids
  - Fluid balance charts
- Infusion devices
  - Gravity devices
  - Pumped systems
  - Patient controlled analgesia (PCA)
  - Anaesthesia pumps
  - Pumps for ambulatory use
  - Infusion device classification

KEY POINTS

IV infusion therapy

- IV infusions are a common sight on hospital wards, and the majority of patients will have IV infusions as a part of their treatment – it is important to have an understanding of the fluid requirements of patients and how fluid regimes are decided.
- Water has an important role in the normal function of the body and fluid balance is a balance between intake and loss.
- Intake is from the normal diet (food and drink) and loss is mainly due to excretion as urine and faeces. Loss is also from sweat (skin) and water vapour from the lungs. The last two are difficult to measure and so are termed *insensible* losses and are based on approximations.
- Assessing a patient's fluid status in clinical practice is somewhat of an imprecise science; however, several methods are used including *fluid balance charts.*

Infusion fluids

- There are two types of fluid used in replacement therapy:
  - Crystalloids
  - Colloids
- Crystalloids are clear fluids made up of water and electrolytes and can be subdivided into three types depending upon their osmolarity compared to plasma:
  - Isotonic – which have the same osmolarity as plasma

- Hypotonic – which have a lower osmolarity compared to plasma
- Hypertonic – which have a higher osmolarity compared to plasma
- Colloids are solutions that contain large molecules which makes them hypertonic and exert an 'osmotic pull' on the fluid in the interstitial and extracellular spaces.

Fluid balance charts

- A fluid balance chart monitors a patient's fluid status by recording fluid intake and output, usually over a 24-hour period.
- Fluid intake is usually by oral liquid, food, enteral and infusion fluids; output is usually by urine, vomiting, diarrhoea, sweat or via drains.
- At the end of 24 hours, fluid balance is given by the total input taken away from the total output:

$$\text{fluid balance} = \text{total input} - \text{total output}$$

Infusion devices

Various systems are available.

Gravity devices

- These depend entirely on gravity to drive the infusion; flow is measured by counting the drops.
- A gravity device should only be considered for low-risk infusions such as sodium chloride, dextrose saline and dextrose infusions.
- A gravity device should not be used for infusions
  - containing potassium.
  - containing drug therapies requiring accurate monitoring or delivery of accurate volumes.
  - delivered to volume sensitive patients.

Pumped systems

These include the following.

Volumetric pumps

- Preferred pumps for medium and large flow rate and volume infusions, although some are designed specially to operate at low flow rates for neonatal use (not recommended for <5 mL/hour).

Syringe pumps

- These are used to administer drugs or infusions in small or medium volumes, and are calibrated at rates 0.1 to 99 mL/hour (recommended for <5 mL/hour).
- Syringe pumps are used extensively where small volumes of highly concentrated drugs are required at low flow rates – usually in intensive care settings.

Patient-controlled analgesia (PCA) pumps
- These pumps are specifically designed for this purpose and are programmable to tailor analgesia for individual needs.

Anaesthesia pumps
- These are syringe pumps designed for use in anaesthesia or sedation and must be used *only* for this purpose; they are unsuitable for any other use. They should be restricted to operating and high dependency areas.

Pumps for ambulatory use
- Ambulatory pumps can be carried around by patients whether they are in hospital or at home.
- The most common type is a syringe driver, and this is typically used for pain.

IV INFUSION THERAPY

- IV infusions are a common sight on hospital wards, and the majority of patients will have IV infusions as a part of their treatment.
- IV fluids should not be considered simply as a means of administering drugs or as plasma expanders. Inappropriate use can lead to imbalances in electrolytes, acid-base disturbances and fluid imbalances.
- As nurses administer IV fluids on a regular basis, it is important to have an understanding of the fluid requirements of patients and how fluid regimes are decided.
- Water has an important role in the normal function of the body. Its major function is as a transport system for nutrients and waste products. Also the kidneys require a minimum of 500 to 700 mL to maintain normal renal function, and the lung surface must be 'wet' to allow gaseous exchange. Water is also important in the maintenance of blood volume. Therefore, it is important to maintain an adequate fluid balance.
- A correct balance of electrolytes (such as sodium, potassium, magnesium and calcium) is important in electric conduction and muscle contraction.

Fluid balance in man
- It is a balance between intake and loss (Figure 9.1).
- Intake is from the normal diet (food and drink), and loss is mainly due to excretion as urine and faeces. Loss is also from sweat (skin) and water vapour from the lungs. The last two are difficult to measure and so are termed *insensible* losses and are based on approximations.

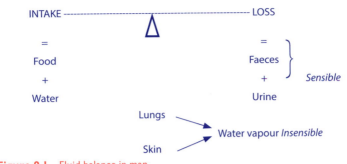

Figure 9.1   Fluid balance in man.

- It is difficult to predict the daily water loss for an average man since there can be a large range in the water loss per day. However, average water loss per day is shown in the following table.

	RANGE	AVERAGE DAILY LOSSES	
Insensible losses			
Skin	400–500 mL/day	450 mL/day	18%
Lungs	300–600 mL/day	400 mL/day	16%
Sensible losses			
Faeces	100–200 mL/day	150 mL/day	6%
Urine	500–3,000 mL/day	1,500 mL/day	60%
Totals		**2,500 mL/day**	**100%**

- It is accepted that the daily loss is around 2,500 mL per day. Obviously, this can only be used as a guide; several factors can alter daily losses.
- In the unwell patient, there may be increased intake via IV fluids, but more importantly, there may be increased loss through diarrhoea/vomiting, pyrexia, fistula/drains and increased diuresis. Conversely, there may be reduced oral intake and reduced output due to renal impairment.
- The body tries to maintain a balance between intake and loss by making internal adjustments (homeostasis) – the details are beyond the scope of this book; the reader should consult relevant articles or pharmacology texts.
- Assessing a patient's fluid status in clinical practice is somewhat of an imprecise science; however, several methods are used to build a wider picture:
  - Patient history
  - Clinical examination of the patient

- Fluid balance charts
- Weighing the patient
- Blood biochemistry

Infusion fluids

- There are two types of fluid used in replacement therapy:
  - Crystalloids
  - Colloids
- Crystalloids are clear fluids made up of water and electrolytes and can be subdivided into three types depending upon their osmolarity compared to plasma:
  - Isotonic – which have the same osmolarity as plasma, e.g. sodium chloride 0.9%, sodium chloride 0.18%/glucose 4%, glucose 5%, Hartmann's
  - Hypotonic – which have a lower osmolarity compared to plasma, e.g. sodium chloride 0.45%
  - Hypertonic – which have a higher osmolarity compared to plasma, e.g. sodium chloride 3%, glucose 10%, sodium chloride 0.45%/glucose 5%
- Colloids do not contain any electrolytes but are solutions that contain large molecules that do not readily leave the intravascular space. This makes them hypertonic and they exert an 'osmotic pull' on the fluid in the interstitial and extracellular spaces. Examples include gelatins.

Fluid balance charts

- A fluid balance chart monitors a patient's fluid status by recording fluid intake and output, usually over a 24-hour period.
- Fluid intake is usually by oral liquid, food, enteral and infusion fluids; output is usually by urine, vomiting, diarrhoea, sweat or via drains.
- Accurate measurement not only is linked to the NMC essential skills clusters, it is also important in identifying patients at risk of dehydration or fluid overload.
- At the end of 24 hours, fluid balance is given by the total input taken away from the total output:

fluid balance = total input – total output

Running or cumulative totals

- Although maintaining a fluid balance chart is simply adding or subtracting numbers, some numeracy skill may be needed when dealing with negative numbers – especially if a running or cumulative total is being kept. Working with negative numbers should not be as daunting as it first seems:

- If adding two negative numbers together, simply add them together. For example, adding –300 mL and –500 mL, the answer is –800 mL.
- However, if adding a negative and a positive number together, subtraction occurs. Consider +300 mL and –500 mL, the answer is –200 mL (500 – 300 = 200); the larger number is negative so the answer is negative.
- Now consider –300 mL and +500 mL, the answer is +200 mL (500 – 300 = 200); the larger number is positive so the answer is positive.

Example

	INPUT					OUTPUT					
	ORAL	IVT SUB CUT	IV DRUGS	NG/ PEG/ TPN	TOTAL INPUT	URINE	NGT/ VOMIT	BOWEL/ STOMA	DRAIN/ OTHER	TOTAL OUTPUT	RUNNING TOTAL
08:00	150 ml				150 ml						+150 ml
09:00						250 ml				250 ml	–100 ml
10:00	200 ml				350 ml						+100 ml
11:00	150 ml				500 ml	200 ml				450 ml	+50 ml
12:00									300 ml		–250 ml

- Fluid balance charts may vary between hospitals but essentially measure fluid input and output over a 24-hour period, probably keeping a running total so that fluid status can be determined at any time.
- The following is no meant to show how to complete a chart, but merely to illustrate the arithmetic to do so.

Example

	INPUT					OUTPUT					
	ORAL	IVT SUB CUT	IV DRUGS	NG/ PEG/ TPN	TOTAL INPUT	URINE	NGT/ VOMIT	BOWEL/ STOMA	DRAIN/ OTHER	TOTAL OUTPUT	RUNNING TOTAL
08:00	150 ml				150 ml						+150 ml
09:00						250 ml				250 ml	–100 ml
10:00	200 ml				350 ml						+100 ml
11:00	150 ml	125 ml			625 ml	200 ml				450 ml	+175 ml
12:00		125 ml			750 ml						+300 ml
13:00	150 ml	125 ml			1,025 ml	180 ml				630 ml	+395 ml

Continued

	INPUT				OUTPUT					
	ORAL	IVT SUB CUT	IV DRUGS	NG/ PEG/ TPN	TOTAL INPUT	URINE	NGT/ VOMIT	BOWEL/ STOMA	DRAIN/ OTHER	TOTAL OUTPUT	RUNNING TOTAL
14:00		125 ml			1,150 ml						+520 ml
15:00	150 ml	125 ml			1,425 ml						+795 ml
16:00		125 ml			1,550 ml						+920 ml
17:00		125 ml			1,675 ml	150 ml				780 ml	+895 ml
18:00	150 ml	125 ml			1,950 ml						+1,170 ml
19:00						120 ml				900 ml	+1,050 ml
20:00											+1,050 ml
21:00	150 ml				2,100 ml						+1,200 ml
22:00						250 ml				1,150 ml	+950 ml
23:00											+950 ml
00:00											+950 ml
01:00											+950 ml
02:00											+950 ml
03:00											+950 ml
04:00											+950 ml
05:00											+950 ml
06:00											+950 ml
07:00											+950 ml
TOTAL					2,100 ml					1,150 ml	
								Balance 950 ml			

A 1 L infusion of sodium chloride 0.9% was started at 11:00 for 8 hours (125 mL per hour for 8 hours).

Total input = 2,100 mL
Total output = 1,150 mL
fluid balance = total input − total output
2,100 mL − 1,150 mL = 950 mL

Patient one

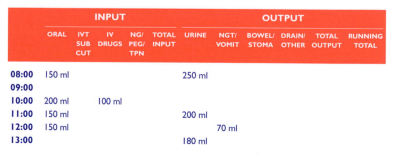

	INPUT				OUTPUT					
	ORAL	IVT SUB CUT	IV DRUGS	NG/ PEG/ TPN	TOTAL INPUT	URINE	NGT/ VOMIT	BOWEL/ STOMA	DRAIN/ OTHER	TOTAL OUTPUT	RUNNING TOTAL
08:00	150 ml					250 ml					
09:00											
10:00	200 ml		100 ml								
11:00	150 ml					200 ml					
12:00	150 ml						70 ml				
13:00						180 ml					

Continued

| | INPUT | | | | | OUTPUT | | | | | |
	ORAL	IVT SUB CUT	IV DRUGS	NG/ PEG/ TPN	TOTAL INPUT	URINE	NGT/ VOMIT	BOWEL/ STOMA	DRAIN/ OTHER	TOTAL OUTPUT	RUNNING TOTAL
14:00			100 ml								
15:00	150 ml										
16:00						150 ml					
17:00											
18:00	150 ml		100 ml						250 ml		
19:00	200 ml					100 ml					
20:00											
21:00	150 ml										
22:00			100 ml								
23:00						250 ml					
00:00											
01:00											
02:00											
03:00											
04:00											
05:00											
06:00											
07:00											
Total											
						Balance					

Try to answer the following questions:

1. What time did the FBC start?
2. What happened at 12:00?
3. How much urine had voided by 16:00?
4. What was the total input and output?
5. What was the final balance?

Patient two

| | INPUT | | | | | OUTPUT | | | | | |
	ORAL	IVT SUB CUT	IV DRUGS	NG/ PEG/ TPN	TOTAL INPUT	URINE	NGT/ VOMIT	BOWEL/ STOMA	DRAIN/ OTHER	TOTAL OUTPUT	RUNNING TOTAL
08:00	150 ml					300 ml					
09:00											
10:00	200 ml					100 ml					
11:00	150 ml										
12:00	150 ml					200 ml					
13:00		125 ml									
14:00	200 ml	125 ml				150 ml					

Continued

	INPUT					OUTPUT					
	ORAL	IVT SUB CUT	IV DRUGS	NG/ PEG/ TPN	TOTAL INPUT	URINE	NGT/ VOMIT	BOWEL/ STOMA	DRAIN/ OTHER	TOTAL OUTPUT	RUNNING TOTAL
15:00	150 ml	125 ml									
16:00		125 ml					80 ml				
17:00											
18:00	150 ml					350 ml					
19:00	200 ml										
20:00											
21:00	150 ml										
22:00											
23:00						250 ml					
00:00											
01:00											
02:00											
03:00											
04:00											
05:00											
06:00											
07:00											
Total											
							Balance				

Try to answer the following questions:

1. What time did the FBC start?
2. What happened at 18:00?
3. How much urine had voided by 16:00?
4. What was the total input and output?
5. What was the final balance?

Patient three

	INPUT					OUTPUT					
	ORAL	IVT SUB CUT	IV DRUGS	NG/ PEG/ TPN	TOTAL INPUT	URINE	NGT/ VOMIT	BOWEL/ STOMA	DRAIN/ OTHER	TOTAL OUTPUT	RUNNING TOTAL
08:00	150 ml					250 ml					
09:00											
10:00	200 ml		500 ml						450 ml		
11:00						200 ml					
12:00	150 ml										
13:00						180 ml					
14:00											
15:00	150 ml		500 ml								

Continued

	INPUT				OUTPUT					
	ORAL	IVT SUB CUT	IV DRUGS	NG/ PEG/ TPN	TOTAL INPUT	URINE	NGT/ VOMIT	BOWEL/ STOMA	DRAIN/ OTHER	TOTAL OUTPUT	RUNNING TOTAL
16:00						150 ml					
17:00											
18:00									250 ml		
19:00						100 ml					
20:00			500 ml								
21:00	150 ml										
22:00	150 ml										
23:00						250 ml					
00:00											
01:00											
02:00											
03:00											
04:00											
05:00											
06:00											
07:00											
Total											
								Balance			

Try to answer the following questions:

1. What time did the FBC start?
2. What happened at 15:00?
3. How much urine had voided by 19:00?
4. What was the total input and output?
5. What was the final balance?

ANSWERS

Patient one

	INPUT				OUTPUT					
	ORAL	IVT SUB CUT	IV DRUGS	NG/ PEG/ TPN	TOTAL INPUT	URINE	NGT/ VOMIT	BOWEL/ STOMA	DRAIN/ OTHER	TOTAL OUTPUT	RUNNING TOTAL
08:00	150 ml				150 ml	250 ml				250 ml	−100 ml
09:00											−100 ml
10:00	200 ml		100 ml		450 ml						+200 ml
11:00	150 ml				600 ml	200 ml				450 ml	+150 ml
12:00	150 ml				750 ml		70 ml			520 ml	+230 ml
13:00						180 ml				700 ml	+50 ml

Continued

	INPUT					OUTPUT					
	ORAL	IVT SUB CUT	IV DRUGS	NG/ PEG/ TPN	TOTAL INPUT	URINE	NGT/ VOMIT	BOWEL/ STOMA	DRAIN/ OTHER	TOTAL OUTPUT	RUNNING TOTAL
14:00			100 ml		850 ml						+150 ml
15:00	150 ml				1,000 ml						+300 ml
16:00						150 ml				850 ml	+150 ml
17:00											+150 ml
18:00	150 ml		100 ml		1,250 ml				250 ml	1,100 ml	+150 ml
19:00	200 ml				1,450 ml	100 ml				1,200 ml	+250 ml
20:00											+250 ml
21:00	150 ml				1,600 ml						+400 ml
22:00			100 ml		1,700 ml						+500 ml
23:00						250 ml				1,450 ml	+250 ml
00:00											+250 ml
01:00											+250 ml
02:00											+250 ml
03:00											+250 ml
04:00											+250 ml
05:00											+250 ml
06:00											+250 ml
07:00											+250 ml
Total					1,700 ml					1,450 ml	
							Balance	250 ml			

1. What time did the FBC start?

     8:00

2. What happened at 12:00?

     Input = 150 mL, output = 70 mL, and running total = +230 mL

3. How much urine had voided by 16:00?

     780 mL (250 + 200 + 180 + 150)

4. What was the total input and output?

     Input = 1,700 mL (150 + 200 + 100 + 150 + 150 + 100 + 150 + 150
     + 100 + 200 + 150 + 100)
     Output = 1,450 mL (250 + 200 + 70 + 180 + 150 + 250 + 100 + 250)

5. What was the final balance?

     250 mL (1,700 − 1,450)

Patient two

	INPUT					OUTPUT					
	ORAL	IVT SUB CUT	IV DRUGS	NG/ PEG/ TPN	TOTAL INPUT	URINE	NGT/ VOMIT	BOWEL/ STOMA	DRAIN/ OTHER	TOTAL OUTPUT	RUNNING TOTAL
08:00	150 ml				150 ml	300 ml				300 ml	−150 ml
09:00											−150 ml
10:00	200 ml				350 ml	100 ml				400 ml	−50 ml
11:00	150 ml				500 ml						+100 ml
12:00	150 ml				650 ml	200 ml				600 ml	+50 ml
13:00		125 ml			775 ml						175 ml
14:00	200 ml	125 ml			1,100 ml	150 ml				750 ml	+350 ml
15:00	150 ml	125 ml			1,375 ml						+625 ml
16:00		125 ml			1,500 ml		80 ml			830 ml	+670 ml
17:00											+670 ml
18:00	150 ml				1,650 ml	350 ml				1,180 ml	+470 ml
19:00	200 ml				1,850 ml						+670 ml
20:00											+670 ml
21:00	150 ml				2,000 ml						+820 ml
22:00											+820 ml
23:00						250 ml				1,430 ml	+570 ml
00:00											+570 ml
01:00											+570 ml
02:00											+570 ml
03:00											+570 ml
04:00											+570 ml
05:00											+570 ml
06:00											+570 ml
07:00											+570 ml
Total					2,000 ml					1,430 ml	
						Balance	570 ml				

1. What time did the FBC start?

   8:00

2. What happened at 18:00?

   Input = 150 mL, output = 350 mL, and running total = +470 mL

3. How much urine had voided by 16:00?

   750 mL (300 + 100 + 200 + 150)

4. What was the total input and output?

   Input = 2,000 mL (150 + 200 + 150 + 150 + 125 + 200 + 125 + 150 + 125 + 125 + 150 + 200 + 150)
   Output = 1,430 mL (300 + 100 + 200 + 150 + 80 + 350 + 250)

5. What was the final balance?

    420 mL (1,850 – 1,430)

Patient three

	INPUT					OUTPUT					
	ORAL	IVT SUB CUT	IV DRUGS	NG/ PEG/ TPN	TOTAL INPUT	URINE	NGT/ VOMIT	BOWEL/ STOMA	DRAIN/ OTHER	TOTAL OUTPUT	RUNNING TOTAL
08:00	150 ml				150 ml	250 ml				250 ml	−100 ml
09:00											−100 ml
10:00	200 ml		500 ml		850 ml				450 ml	700 ml	+150 ml
11:00						200 ml				900 ml	−50 ml
12:00	150 ml				1,000 ml						+100 ml
13:00						180 ml				1,080 ml	−80 ml
14:00											−80 ml
15:00	150 ml		500 ml		1,650 ml						+570 ml
16:00						150 ml				1,230 ml	+420 ml
17:00											+420 ml
18:00									250 ml	1,480 ml	+170 ml
19:00						100 ml				1,580 ml	+70 ml
20:00			500 ml		2,150 ml						+570 ml
21:00	150 ml				2,300 ml						+720 ml
22:00	150 ml				2,450 ml						+870 ml
23:00						250 ml				1,830 ml	+620 ml
00:00											+620 ml
01:00											+620 ml
02:00											+620 ml
03:00											+620 ml
04:00											+620 ml
05:00											+620 ml
06:00											+620 ml
07:00											+620 ml
Total					2,450 ml					1,830 ml	
							Balance	620 ml			

1. What time did the FBC start?

    8:00

2. What happened at 15:00?

    Input = 650 mL (150 + 500) and running total = +570 mL

3. How much urine had voided by 19:00?

    880 mL (250 + 200 + 180 + 150 + 100)

4. What was the total input and output?

Input = 2,450 mL (150 + 200 + 500 + 150 + 150 + 500 + 500 + 150 + 150)
Output = 1,830 mL (250 + 450 + 200 + 180 + 150 + 250 + 100 + 250)

5. What was the final balance?

620 mL (2,450 − 1,830)

INFUSION DEVICES

This is a brief overview of infusion devices available and their use in drug administration. For advice on setting up and using infusion devices and problems associated with them, the reader is advised to seek more detailed references and the manufacturers' manuals.

In general, infusion pumps are capable of accurate delivery of solution over a wide range of volumes and flow rates, and may be designed for specialist application, e.g. for neonatal use.

Gravity devices

Drip rate controllers look like a pump but have no pumping mechanism. These depend entirely on gravity to drive the infusion; the pressure for the infusion depends on the height of the liquid above the infusion site. They use standard solution sets and flow is measured by counting the drops. A drop sensor, attached to the drip chamber of the administration set, monitors the drip rate.

A gravity device should only be considered for low-risk infusions such as sodium chloride, dextrose saline and dextrose infusions. A gravity device *should not* be used for infusions containing potassium, or drug therapies requiring accurate monitoring or delivery of accurate volumes. Infusions, even low risk, should not be delivered to volume sensitive patients via a gravity line but must be given via an infusion pump.

Pumped systems

Volumetric or syringe pumps are the most common.

Volumetric pumps

These pumps are the preferred choice for medium and large volume intravenous or enteral infusions, although some are designed specifically to operate at low flow rates for neonatal use. The rate is given in millilitres per hour (typical range 1–999 mL/hour).

Typically, most volumetric pumps will perform satisfactorily at rates down to 5 mL/hour. A syringe pump should be used for rates lower than 5 mL/hour or when short-term accuracy is required. Volumetric pumps are most suited to administering fluids in categories B and C and at higher flow rates.

All volumetric pumps are designed to use a specific giving set. Using any set other than the correct one will result in reduced accuracy and poor alarm responses. Volumetric pumps must be configured correctly for the specific set.

Delivery of low-risk infusions should be considered via a gravity device rather than a volumetric pump, unless accurate monitoring is required, or the patient is at risk of fluid overload.

Syringe pumps

These are used to administer drugs or infusions in small or medium volumes, and are calibrated for delivery in millilitres per hour, typically 0.1 to 99 mL/hour. Syringe pumps have better short-term accuracy than volumetric pumps and are therefore typically more superior when delivering drugs at rates below 5 mL/hour. Syringe pumps are used extensively where small volumes of highly concentrated drugs are required at low flow rates – usually in intensive care settings.

Patient-controlled analgesia (PCA) pumps

These pumps are specifically designed for this purpose. PCA pumps are typically syringe pumps, as the total volume of drug infused can usually be contained in a single-use syringe. The difference between a PCA pump and a normal syringe pump is that patients are able to deliver a bolus dose themselves. Immediately after delivery the pump will refuse to deliver another bolus until a pre-set time has passed. The pre-set bolus size and lockout time, along with background (constant drug infusion) are pre-programmed by the doctor.

Once programmed, access to the control of the pump is usually restricted. A feature of most PCA pumps is a memory log, which enables the clinician to determine when, and how often, the patient has made a demand and what total volume of drug has been infused over a given time.

Anaesthesia pumps

These are syringe pumps designed for use in anaesthesia or sedation and must be used *only* for this purpose; they are unsuitable for any other use. They should be restricted to operating and high dependency areas. They should be clearly labelled 'Anaesthesia Pump' and restricted to operating theatres and high dependency areas.

Pumps for ambulatory use

Ambulatory pumps have been designed to allow patients to continue receiving treatment or therapy away from a hospital, thereby leading a normal life during treatment. The size and design of these pumps means patients can carry them around in a form of holster. These are miniature versions of syringe pumps which are battery driven. They deliver their dose in bursts, not in an even flow rate, almost like a continual sequence of micro boluses.

Therapies that can be administered by ambulatory pumps include analgesia, continuous and PCA, antibiotic or antiviral infusions, chemotherapy, and hormone delivery.

Syringe drivers

These pumps are designed to deliver drugs accurately over a certain period of time (usually 24 hours). They have the advantage of being small and compact, can be carried easily by the patient, and avoid the need for numerous injections throughout the day. An electronically controlled motor drives the plastic syringe plunger, infusing the syringe contents into the patient.

Various devices suitable for continuous subcutaneous infusion are available. It is not possible to give details of them all here. Most are battery operated but may differ in their method of operation, particularly for setting the delivery rate.

Depending on the pumping mechanism, rates of flow range between 0.01 and 1,000 mL/hour is possible. Delivery rates can be set in millimetres of syringe travel per hour or day, millilitres of fluid per hour or day, or dose units. Some can also be programmed for different delivery modes.

The SIMS Graseby syringe drivers type MS16A (blue panel) and type MS26 (green panel), are described here because they are widely used. This does not imply that these two models are any better than the others. It should be noted that syringe drivers are undergoing continual development and improvement.

There are two types of Graseby syringe drivers:

- MS16A (blue panel) – designed to deliver drugs at an hourly rate
- MS26 (green panel) – designed to deliver drugs at a daily rate (i.e. over 24 hours)

To avoid confusion between the two pumps, the MS16A is clearly marked with a pink 1HR in the bottom right-hand corner; the MS26 has an orange/brown 24HR instead. Rate is set in terms of millimetres per hour or millimetres per day, that is, linear travel of syringe plunger against time.

Calculation of dose

The amount required is the total dose to be given over 24 hours:

1. If the dose is prescribed as 'mg/hour', then it is necessary to calculate the total amount for 24 hours by multiplying by 24, e.g. if the dose is 3 mg/hour, then:
   Total amount required for 24 hours = 3 × 24 = 72 mg.

2. If the dose is prescribed every 4 hours (or whatever), multiply the dose by the number of times the dose is given in 24 hours, i.e. if the dose is 20 mg every 4 hours.

> The dose is being given 6 times in 24 hours (divide 24 by the dosing frequency, i.e. 24/4 = 6).
> Total amount required for 24 hours = 20 × 6 = 120 mg.

3. If the dose is prescribed as 'mg/day' (24 hours), then no calculation is necessary, i.e. if the dose is 60 mg/day (24 hours), then:

> Total amount required for 24 hours = 60 mg.

To set the rate

Always set up a syringe driver to make L about 50 mm with diluent before priming the infusion set. Priming will take about 2 mm of this total, leaving 48 mm of fluid to be transfused over 24 hours. This makes the arithmetic of setting easier. When infusions do not require a priming volume, L should be set at 48 mm. The volume varies from one brand of syringe to another, but the dose and the distance L are the important factors not the volume (Figure 9.2).

MAKE SURE THAT THE INFUSION DEVICE IS SET UP PROPERLY.

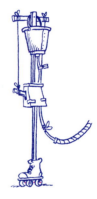

MS16A (blue panel) – mm/hr

$$\text{set rate} = \frac{\text{distance } L \text{ in mm (48)}}{\text{infusion time in hours}}$$

$$\text{For example } \frac{48 \text{ mm}}{24 \text{ hr}} = 2 \text{ mm/hr}$$

So the dial should read: 02 mm/hr.

MS26 (green panel) – mm/24 hours

$$\text{set rate} = \frac{\text{distance } L \text{ in mm (48)}}{\text{infusion time in day}} \quad \text{For example } \frac{48 \text{ mm}}{1 \text{ day}} = 48 \text{ mm/day (24 hours)}$$

So the dial should read: 48 mm/24 hours.

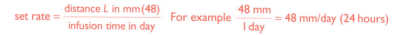

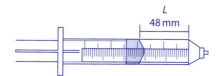

Figure 9.2   Measurement of fluid length (*L*) in syringe.

INFUSION DEVICE CLASSIFICATION

The Medicines and Healthcare Products Regulatory Agency (MHRA) has made recommendations on the safety and performance of infusion devices in order to enable users to make the appropriate choice of equipment to suit most applications. The classification system has been divided into three major categories according to the potential risks involved. A pump suited to the high-risk category of therapy (A) can be safely used for the other categories (B and C). A pump suited to category B can be used for B and C, whereas a pump with the lowest specification (C) is suited only to category C therapies.

Hospitals are required to label each infusion pump with its category, and it will be necessary to know the category of the proposed therapy and match it with a pump of the same or better category.

THERAPY CATEGORY	THERAPY DESCRIPTION	PATIENT GROUP	CRITICAL PERFORMANCE PARAMETERS
A	Drugs with narrow therapeutic margin	Any	Good long-term accuracy
	Drugs with short half-life (5 minutes or less)	Any	Good short-term accuracy
	Any infusion given to neonates	Neonates	Rapid alarm after occlusion
			Small occlusion bolus
			Able to detect very small air embolus (volumetric pumps only)
			Small flow rate increments
			Good bolus accuracy
			Rapid start-up time (syringe pumps only)
B	Drugs, other than those with a short half-life	Any except neonates	Good long-term accuracy
			Alarm after occlusion
	Total parenteral nutrition (TPN)	Volume sensitive except neonates	Small occlusion bolus
			Able to detect small air embolus (volumetric pumps only)
	Fluid maintenance		
	Transfusions		Small flow rate increments
	Diamorphine	Any except neonates	Bolus accuracy

Continued

THERAPY CATEGORY	THERAPY DESCRIPTION	PATIENT GROUP	CRITICAL PERFORMANCE PARAMETERS
C	TPN Fluid maintenance Transfusions	Any except volume sensitive or neonates	Long-term accuracy Alarm after occlusion Small occlusion bolus Able to detect air embolus (volumetric pumps only) Incremental flow rates

Errors involving the incorrect setting of IV pumps are among the most common errors reported. These errors involve volumetric infusion pumps as well as syringe driver and patient-controlled analgesic pumps. Due to the wide variety of uses for these devices, errors in setting the correct drug administration rates may involve narcotic analgesics, insulin, heparin, cardiovascular drugs, and cancer chemotherapy agents. Although a fault with the equipment is frequently cited, testing the pumps after an error has occurred rarely shows that they are in fact faulty. In the vast majority of cases the fault is due to operator error.

It is important that calculations involving dosing and setting infusion rates are checked before using any infusion device.

10 ACTION AND ADMINISTRATION OF MEDICINES

OBJECTIVES

At the end of this chapter, you should be familiar with the following:

- Pharmacokinetics
  - Absorption
  - Distribution
  - Metabolism
  - Elimination
- Pharmacodynamics
- Administration of medicines
  - Oral
  - Parenteral
- Promoting the safer use of injectable medicines

KEY POINTS

In order for a drug to reach its site of action and have an effect, it needs to enter the bloodstream. This is influenced by the route of administration and how the drug is absorbed.

Pharmacokinetics

Pharmacokinetics examines the way in which the body 'handles drugs' and looks at:

- Absorption of drugs into the body
- Distribution around the body
- Elimination or excretion

Pharmacodynamics

This is the study of the mode of action of drugs – how they exert their effect.

Administration of medicines

Which route of administration?

The route of administration depends upon:

- Which is the most convenient route for the patient;
- The drug and its properties;
- The formulations available;
- How quick an effect is required;
- Whether a local or systemic effect is required;
- Clinical condition of the patient – the oral route may not be possible; and
- Whether the patient is compliant or not.

Oral administration

For most patients, the oral route is the most convenient and acceptable way for taking medicines. Drugs may be given as tablets, capsules, or liquids: other means include buccal or sublingual administration.

Parenteral administration

This is the injection of drugs directly into the blood or tissues. The three most common methods are intravenous (IV), subcutaneous (SC), and intramuscular (IM).

Promoting the safer use of injectable medicines

The risks associated with using injectable medicines in clinical areas have been recognized and well known for some time. Recent research evidence indicates that the incidence of errors in prescribing, preparing, and administering injectable medicines is higher than for other forms of medicine. As a consequence, the National Patient Safety Agency (NPSA) issued safety alert 20 – *Promoting Safer Use of Injectable Medicines* – in March 2007. The alert covers multiprofessional safer practice standards with particular emphasis on prescribing, preparation and administration of injectable medicines in clinical areas.

ACTION AND ADMINISTRATION OF MEDICINES

The administration of medicines is a major part of nursing care in various settings. It is important that nurses understand the effect different drugs have in the body.

Not only should newly registered nurses have a basic knowledge of pharmacology, it is essential that nurse prescribers do as well. Nurse prescribers will have to choose which drug to prescribe, and what is most appropriate for the patient – factors such as age (especially the extremes of life), comorbidity, concurrent illness (e.g. dehydration) and choice of pharmaceutical formulation (Young, Weeks, and Hutton 2012) must be considered. All of these factors influence whether a suitable amount of drug reaches the appropriate site of action to have the desired effect.

A pharmacological knowledge will ensure that drugs are correctly administered and that the patient is involved in his or her treatment options and receives the correct information (Lawson and Hennefer 2010).

The NMC Essential Skills Cluster or ESC (NMC 2010), Medicines Management (36) states: 'People can trust the newly registered graduate nurse to ensure safe and effective practice in medicines management through comprehensive knowledge of medicines, their actions, risks and benefits.'

Entry of qualified nurses and midwives to the register

- Applies knowledge of basic pharmacology, how medicines act and interact in the systems of the body, and their therapeutic action.
- Understands common routes and techniques of medicine administration including absorption, metabolism, adverse reactions and interactions.
- Safely manages drug administration and monitors effects.*
- Reports adverse incidents and near misses.
- Safely manages anaphylaxis.

In order to achieve this, knowledge of the following is recommended:

- Related anatomy and physiology
- Drug pathways and how medicines act
- Impacts of physiological state of patients on drug responses and safety, for example, the older adult, children and pregnant or breastfeeding women, and significant pathologies such as renal or hepatic impairments
- Pharmacodynamics – the effects of drugs and their mechanisms of action in the body
- Pharmacotherapeutics – the therapeutic actions of certain medicines; risks versus benefits of medication
- Pharmacokinetics and how doses are determined by dynamics and systems in the body

INTRODUCTION

The aim of this section of the book is to look at the administration of medicines with the emphasis on applying the principles learned during drug calculations.

In order for a drug to reach its site of action and have the intended effect, it needs to enter the bloodstream. This is influenced by the route of administration and how the drug is absorbed.

If you are prescribing (or administering) medicines, you should understand how drugs work and interact with the body. To facilitate your understanding, we will look at:

- Pharmacokinetics (how the body deals with drugs) and pharmacodynamics (how drugs have an effect on the body)
- Common routes of administration
- Source and interpretation of drug information

---

* An ESC where skills in numeracy and calculation have been identified.

PHARMACOKINETICS AND PHARMACODYNAMICS

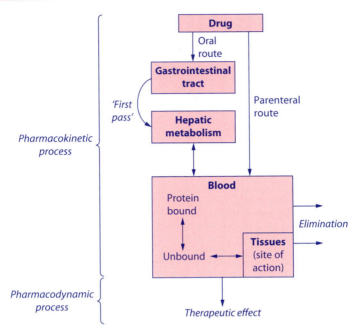

Figure 10.1 The pharmacokinetic and pharmacodynamic processes.

Pharmacokinetics

The following is a brief introduction to a complex subject. Pharmacokinetics will enable you to understand some of the science behind the safe and efficacious management of medicines. The aim is to provide a general idea of the processes involved in order to ensure medicines are safe and effective, and also to explain some of the terms frequently used.

If a drug is going to have an effect in the body it needs to be present:

- In the right place
- At the right concentration
- For the right amount of time

Pharmacokinetics examines the way in which the body handles drugs and looks at:

- Absorption of drugs into the body
- Distribution around the body

- Metabolism which is the breakdown of a drug by the body
- Elimination or excretion

The mnemonic ADME is used to remember these four processes.

Pharmacokinetics is an active (kinetic) process in which all the above occur at the same time. Knowing about the pharmacokinetics of a drug allows us to determine:

- What dose to give
- How often to give it
- How to change the dose in certain medical conditions
- How some drug interactions occur

Absorption

For a drug to be absorbed it needs to enter the systemic circulation. The oral route is the most commonly used and convenient method of administration for drugs. When given orally, the drug passes into the intestines via the stomach – during this passage, the drug is absorbed.

Drugs must be relatively stable to the acid environment of the stomach – some drugs are degraded by the acid content of the gastro-intestinal (GI) tract and therefore cannot be given orally, e.g. insulin. However, some drugs are formulated in such a way to be administered orally, e.g. enteric-coated (EC) drugs.

So how is a drug absorbed orally? Most drugs are absorbed by diffusion through the wall of the intestine into the bloodstream. In order to achieve this, the drug needs to pass through a cell membrane.

The GI tract has a very large surface area where drugs can be absorbed. Any situation that reduces this absorptive area, e.g. inflammatory bowel disease or surgery, can decrease the absorption of drugs.

Drugs diffuse across cell membranes from a region of high concentration (GI tract) to one of low concentration (blood). The rate of diffusion depends not only upon these differences in concentration, but also on the physiochemical properties of the drug.

Cell membranes have a lipid or fatty layer, so drugs that can dissolve in this layer (lipid soluble) can pass through easily. Drugs that are not lipid soluble will not pass readily across the cell membrane. However, some drugs are transported across the cell membrane by carrier proteins (facilitated diffusion) or actively transported across by a pump system (active transport).

Most absorption occurs in the small intestine, which has a very good blood supply – one reason why most absorption occurs in this part of the gut. Anything that delays or speeds up the drug reaching the intestines can affect the rate and amount of drug absorbed, e.g. food, other drugs and gut motility.

Food in the stomach slows down the progress of a drug through the GI tract by slowing down the rate at which the GI tract empties (gastric motility or emptying time). In addition, certain foods may interact with the drug reducing the amount available, e.g. milk and tetracyclines. These are the reasons certain drugs are given before food.

Antacids can increase or decrease the rate at which a drug is absorbed, or the total amount absorbed. Antacids change the acid environment (raise the pH) which can affect the way a drug dissolves (dissolution); delay gastric emptying; and interact making less drug available to be absorbed.

Gastric motility can be increased if the patient has diarrhoea or takes certain drugs, e.g. metoclopramide. Vomiting can also affect the absorption of drugs.

Bioavailability
Bioavailability is a term that is used to describe the amount (sometimes referred to as the fraction) of the administered dose that reaches the systemic circulation which is available to have an effect.

The bioavailability of a drug can be affected by:

- How the drug is absorbed
- The extent of drug metabolism before reaching the systemic circulation – known as first-pass metabolism (see later)
- The formulation and manufacture of the drug – this can affect the way a medicine disintegrates and dissolves

The term bioavailability is used generally in reference to drugs given by the oral route, although it can also refer to other routes of administration. Drugs given by intravenous injection are said to have 100% bioavailability when compared to those given orally.

Distribution
After a drug enters the systemic circulation, it is distributed to the body's tissues. The extent and the way a drug is distributed are influenced by a numbers of factors:

- The rate of blood flow to the tissues
- The amount and/or type of tissue
- Blood-brain/placenta barriers
- The way in which blood and tissues interact with each other
- Plasma proteins

Organs that are well perfused (e.g. heart, liver and kidneys) will receive large amounts of drug, whereas tissues that are poorly perfused (e.g. fat, bone and muscle) will receive less drug, and it may take more time for a drug to reach levels to have a therapeutic effect.

The body has mechanisms that prevent chemicals from entering and harming the brain, known as the blood–brain barrier. Psychotropic drugs such as antidepressants must be able to pass into the central nervous system to exert their effect, and as a consequence these drugs are highly lipophilic.

The placental barrier works in a similar way to protect the developing baby.

Plasma protein binding of drugs

The extent to which a drug distributes into tissues depends upon how it binds to proteins found in the plasma and dissolves in the fatty layers of the tissues. Once drugs are present in the bloodstream, they are transported either in solution as free (unbound) drug or reversibly bound to plasma proteins (e.g. albumin, glycoproteins and lipoproteins).

When drugs are bound to plasma proteins they:

- Do not undergo first-pass metabolism as only the unbound drug can be metabolized.
- Have no effect because only the free (unbound) fraction of the drug can enter or distribute into the tissues to exert an effect. This drug-protein complex is too large to cross cell membranes.

As a drug is removed or excreted, the drug-protein complex can separate (or dissociate) to re-establish the ratio (or equilibrium) between free and unbound drug. This process determines the amount of drug, the time spent, and thus efficacy, at the target site (Figure 10.2).

The process of binding is nonspecific and different drugs can compete for the same binding sites. If a highly protein-bound drug already occupies a number of binding sites and another highly protein-bound drug is added, then a situation of competition for binding can arise. This can result in displacement of the original drug causing a higher concentration of free (unbound) drug.

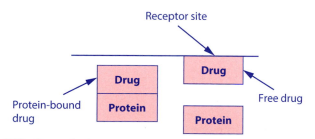

Figure 10.2 Protein binding.

This can be important if the displaced drug has a narrow therapeutic index. The term *narrow therapeutic window* or *index* is used to describe drugs for which the toxic level is only slightly above the therapeutic range, and a slight increase in unbound drug may therefore result in adverse effects. (See later for a more complete explanation of narrow therapeutic window or index.) For example, the anticoagulant warfarin can be displaced by aspirin increasing the amount of free anticoagulant producing a risk of haemorrhage.

If a patient suffers from a condition in which plasma proteins are deficient (e.g. liver disease or malnutrition), the number of binding sites are reduced and there will be more free (unbound) drug available. A normal dose of a drug could then be dangerous, because so little is bound by available protein, thus increasing the availability of unbound drug. The drug then starts to distribute itself around the body and drug metabolism starts.

Volume of distribution

Drugs are distributed unevenly between various body fluids and tissues according to their physical and chemical properties. The term *volume of distribution* is used to reflect the amount of drug left in the bloodstream (plasma) after all the drug has been absorbed and distributed.

If a drug is 'held' in the bloodstream, it will have a small volume of distribution. If very little drug remains in the bloodstream, it has a large volume of distribution. We have to estimate values because we can only measure the drug concentration in the bloodstream and so it is known as the 'apparent' volume of distribution.

The analogy of describing people as 'buckets' is commonly used to illustrate the concept of distribution and clearance. People can be described as large, medium or small buckets.

Imagine that a patient needs a certain amount of drug in order to reach a concentration that will produce the desired effect. In other words, there is a need to 'fill the bucket' (the patient) with the right amount of drug. If the bucket is not filled properly, then the desired effect may not happen. If the bucket is overfilled, then toxicity could occur (i.e. overdose). When a blood level is taken, the amount of drug in the bucket (body) is being measured.

Metabolism

This is the process by which the body modifies or breaks down chemicals (including drugs) allowing eventual elimination from the body. Metabolism of drugs mainly occurs in the liver, but may also occur in the kidneys, intestines, lungs, plasma and placenta. Drugs that are absorbed from the GI tract are transported to the liver via the hepatic portal vein.

The liver is the main site for drug breakdown or metabolism (by liver enzymes), before reaching the general circulation and their sites of action. This removal or modification of a drug, before it is available to have an effect, is called first-pass metabolism or first-pass effect.

Some drugs

- pass through the liver unchanged
- are converted to an inactive form or metabolite which is excreted
- are inactive and are converted to an active form (these are known as pro-drugs)
- produce an active metabolite which has an effect in its own right

As a result of first-pass metabolism, only a fraction of drug may eventually reach the tissues to have a therapeutic effect.

If the drug is given parenterally the liver is bypassed and so the amount of drug that reaches the circulation is greater compared to oral administration. As a consequence, much smaller parenteral doses are needed to produce an equivalent effect. For example, propranolol – if given IV, the dose is 1 mg; if given orally, the dose is 40 mg or higher.

Drugs that are rapidly metabolized will have a short duration of action and therefore need to be given more often. In contrast, drugs that are slowly metabolized can be given less often.

Codeine is a pro-drug and is converted to morphine in the liver. The capacity to metabolize codeine to morphine can vary considerably between individuals. People can be classified as poor, intermediate, extensive or ultra-rapid metabolizers, and this can vary with ethnic origin. There is a marked increase in morphine toxicity in patients who are ultra-rapid codeine metabolizers and a reduced therapeutic effect in poor codeine metabolizers.

A European review (October 2012) was triggered by concerns of an increased risk of morphine toxicity when susceptible children receive codeine for pain after surgery. One of the conclusions was that codeine should be contraindicated in all patients known to be ultra-rapid metabolizers (less than 12 years old). In addition, children (aged below 18 years) who undergo surgery for removal of the tonsils or adenoids should not receive codeine, as these patients are more susceptible to respiratory problems (MHRA 2013).

Enzyme-inducing or -inhibiting drugs

Some drugs increase the activity of enzymes in the liver (enzyme inducers, e.g. carbamazepine) that break down drugs – so a larger dose of affected drug is needed for a therapeutic effect. Other drugs may inhibit or reduce enzyme production (enzyme inhibitors, e.g. erythromycin) which reduces the rate at which another drug is inactivated – so a smaller dose of affected drug is needed for a therapeutic effect. Care must be taken if an enzyme-inducing or -inhibiting drug is stopped – dosing of affected drugs may have to be changed.

Entero-hepatic recycling

The liver can transfer substances, including drugs, either unchanged or as conjugated drug (metabolite), to the gallbladder in bile.

The bile is released in the gut lumen, from which the free drug can be reabsorbed. In the small intestine, bacteria can act on the conjugated drug and free the active drug, which may in turn also be reabsorbed, and enters the portal vein, which carries it back to the liver. This cycle is called the entero-hepatic cycle and may be repeated several times, significantly prolonging the body's exposure to the drug.

The effect of this is to create a 'reservoir' of recirculating drug and prolong its duration of action. Not many drugs undergo this recycling; one example is morphine. However, if the gut bacteria are reduced, e.g. by antibiotics, the drug is not recycled and is lost more quickly.

Drugs secreted into bile will finally pass through to the large intestine and be excreted in the faeces. Liver disease can reduce the ability of the liver to synthesize hepatic enzymes and hence the ability to metabolize drugs (Figure 10.3).

Elimination

There are various routes by which drugs can be eliminated. The most important routes are the kidneys and the liver; the least important are the biliary system, skin, lungs and gut. Drugs are primarily eliminated from the body by a combination of renal excretion (main route) and hepatic metabolism.

Relative importance of metabolism and excretion in drug clearance

Depending upon their properties, some drugs mainly undergo metabolic clearance (liver) or renal clearance. Lipid-soluble drugs can readily cross cell membranes and are more likely to enter liver cells and undergo extensive

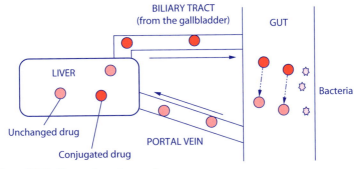

Figure 10.3 Entero-hepatic recycling.

hepatic clearance. However, if a drug is water soluble, it will not be able to enter liver cells easily, so it is more likely to be eliminated by the kidneys.

Only water-soluble drugs are eliminated by the kidneys; lipid-soluble drugs need to be metabolized to water-soluble metabolites before they can be excreted by the kidneys. If a lipid-soluble drug is filtered by the kidneys, it is largely reabsorbed in the tubules. Drugs and/or their metabolites are transported by capillaries to the kidneys.

The excretion of drugs by the kidneys is achieved by two main processes which occur in the nephron of the kidney:

- Glomerular filtration – acts like a sieve, allowing small drugs and those not bound to plasma proteins to filter from the blood to the proximal tubule
- Active secretion (by transport carriers) into the proximal tubule

Some drugs and their metabolites may be reabsorbed back into the bloodstream. This is because water is reabsorbed as a means of conserving body fluid – as this movement occurs, some drugs are transported along with it (see Figure 10.4).

Several factors may affect the rate at which drugs are eliminated by the kidneys:

- Kidney disease and/or renal failure
- Reduced blood flow to the kidneys
- pH of urine – changes can increase excretion
- Molecular weight of drug/metabolite

Going back to the 'bucket' analogy, clearance can be represented by a hole in the bottom of the bucket. In order to keep the bucket (or body) filled with the same amount of drug, it needs to be continuously or periodically re-filled to replace the drug which is lost through the hole.

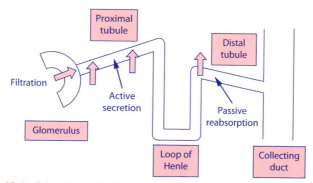

Figure 10.4 Excretion and reabsorption of drugs by the kidney.

Once again, if you replace too much, toxicity can occur; if not enough, then the desired effect may not be achieved.

Blood levels or plasma concentration

After a period of time following administration, a drug will reach its highest level or concentration – denoted as C_{max}. The time taken to reach this level is denoted as T_{max}.

The minimum concentration (denoted C_{min}) is the amount of drug left just before the next dose is administered. The time taken to reach this level is denoted as T_{min}.

Therapeutic window or index

Therapeutic window or index denotes the maximum and minimum levels between which a drug is effective; above the maximum level the drug becomes toxic, and below the minimum, the drug is ineffective (subtherapeutic).

Some drugs are said to have a narrow therapeutic window or index in that the levels between being toxic and ineffective are small (or narrow). Thus small changes in the pharmacokinetics can have a dramatic effect. Examples include carbamazepine, digoxin, gentamicin, lithium, phenytoin and warfarin.

Half-life ($t_{1/2}$)

The duration of action of a drug is sometimes referred to as its half-life. This is the period of time required for the concentration or amount of drug in the body to be reduced by one-half of its original value. We usually consider the half-life of a drug in relation to the amount of the drug in plasma, and this is influenced by the removal of a drug from the plasma (clearance) and the distribution of the drug in the various body tissues (volume of distribution).

Below is an illustration of half-life using 100 mg of drug.

NUMBER OF HALF-LIVES	AMOUNT OF DRUG CLEARED	AMOUNT OF DRUG IN THE BODY
1	50%	50 mg
2	75% (50% + 25%)	25 mg
3	87.5% (50% + 25% + 12.5%)	12.5 mg
4	93.75% (50% + 25% + 12.5% + 6.25%)	6.25 mg
5	96.875% (50% + 25% + 12.5% + 6.25% + 3.125%)	3.125 mg

So you can see that after five half-lives, the majority of a single dose of drug (around 97%) will be lost.

Half-life can also be used to estimate when a drug reaches steady state. When a patient starts to take a drug at regular intervals, the concentration of drug in the body slowly increases until it becomes relatively constant (steady state). As repeated doses are given, a proportion of that dose will remain; all of these proportions (when added together) will contribute to the total concentration (or blood level).

Below is an illustration of half-life using 100 mg of drug.

NUMBER OF HALF-LIVES	DOSE	DOSE PLUS AMOUNT REMAINING FROM THE PREVIOUS DOSE	AMOUNT ELIMINATED	AMOUNT OF DRUG IN THE BODY
1	100 mg	100 mg = 100 mg	50 mg	50 mg
2	100 mg	100 mg + 50 mg = 150 mg	75 mg	75 mg
3	100 mg	100 mg + 75 mg = 175 mg	87.5 mg	87.5 mg
4	100 mg	100 mg + 87.5 mg = 187.5 mg	93.75 mg	93.75 mg
5	100 mg	100 mg + 93.75 mg = 193.75 mg	96.875 mg	96.875 mg

So you can see that approximately after five half-lives, steady-state is reached after repeated dosing.

To be therapeutically effective, drugs that have short half-lives (cleared from the blood rapidly) need to be given frequently in regular doses to build up and maintain a high enough concentration compared to those with longer half-lives, which can be administered less often.

Dosing

Dosing intervals are based on half-life data giving regimens that produce stable blood levels – keeping them below toxic, but above minimum effective levels.

As repeated doses of a drug are administered, its plasma concentration builds up and reaches what is known as a steady state (denoted as Css). This is when the concentration has reached a level that has a therapeutic effect, and as long as regular doses are given to counteract the amount being eliminated, it will continue to have an effect.

The time taken to reach the steady state is about five times the half-life of a drug. Drugs like digoxin and warfarin with a long half-life will take longer to reach a steady state than drugs with a shorter half-life.

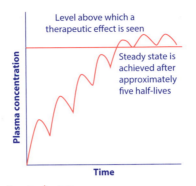

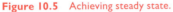

Figure 10.5 Achieving steady state.

Sometimes a loading dose may be administered so that a steady state is reached more quickly, and then smaller 'maintenance' doses are given to ensure that the drug levels stay within the steady state (Figure 10.5).

Estimation of renal function

Renal function in adults is routinely reported on the basis of estimated glomerular filtration rate (eGFR), which is normalized to a body surface area of 1.73 m² and derived from the modification of diet in renal disease (MDRD) formula. It is calculated using serum creatinine concentration, age, sex and ethnic origin.

Published information on the effects of renal impairment on drug elimination is usually stated in terms of creatinine clearance (CrCl) – based on the Cockcroft & Gault (C&G) estimation – as a substitute for glomerular filtration rate (GFR).

Although the two measures of renal function are not interchangeable, in practice, for most drugs and for most patients (over 18 years) of average build and height, eGFR (MDRD) can be used to determine dosage adjustments in place of CrCl (C&G).

The information on dosage adjustment in the British National Formulary (BNF) is usually expressed as eGFR as opposed to CrCl, and this can be used for a large number of drugs and patients.

However, there are exceptions where the absolute GFR or CrCl calculated by the C&G formula should be used:

- Patients at extremes of body weight (BMI <18.5 kg/m² or >30 kg/m²). If using absolute GFR for these patients it may be necessary to base the calculation on ideal body weight.
- Children under 18 years.
- Potentially toxic drugs with a narrow therapeutic index. In the BNF, values for creatinine clearance or another measure of renal function are included where possible.

An individual's absolute glomerular filtration rate can be calculated from the eGFR as follows:

$$GFR_{Absolute} = eGFR \times \left(\frac{\text{individual's body surface area}}{1.73} \right)$$

The BNF is generally not a good resource for dosing patients with renal impairment. It does not make a distinction between steady-state chronic kidney disease (CKD) and acute kidney injury (AKI) – other reference sources are available for information about CKD and AKI. Clinical interpretation is necessary.

Pharmacodynamics

This is the study of the mode of action of drugs – how they exert their effect and mode of action. There are varied and complex physiological systems that control bodily functions (homeostasis). Drugs exert their effect by acting on those physiological systems – they can act on receptors, enzyme systems, ion channels or carrier/transport mechanisms.

Receptors

Receptors are usually proteins found on cell membranes or within a cell on which natural hormones and neurotransmitters can bind to and cause a specific effect.

There are various receptors and subtypes, and it is not fully understood as to how they exert their effect.

In order for a drug to act at a specific receptor site, it must have a complementary structure to the receptor – sometimes referred to as a 'lock and key' action. Drugs can bind to these sites in two ways – cause an effect (agonists) (Figure 10.6) or block an effect (antagonists). Most drugs acting as antagonists work by competing with the normal agonist; their action depends upon the concentration of antagonist versus agonist.

Drugs can act by producing enhanced effects, e.g. salbutamol is a beta-2 receptor agonist producing a bronchodilator effect in asthma by acting on the beta-2 receptors in smooth muscle cells.

Conversely, drugs can act by blocking a response, e.g. ranitidine is an H-2 histamine receptor antagonist. One action of histamine is as a stimulant effect of gastric secretion. Ranitidine can block the action of histamine reducing gastric acid secretion by about 70%.

There is another way in which drugs may act – as partial agonists. A partial agonist does not produce a full effect as an agonist – if there is a high concentration of partial agonists, they may bind to a receptor site without producing an effect. However, in doing so, the partial agonist blocks that receptor to other agonists and so it is acting as an antagonist – so it has a 'dual' action.

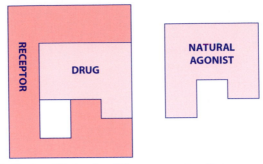

Figure 10.6 'Lock and Key' action of drugs at receptor sites.

Drugs are not always specific to a particular receptor where the desired effect is wanted. They can also act on similar receptors in other areas, producing unwanted effects (side effects).

Enzyme systems

An enzyme is a protein which acts as a catalyst that also controls many body activities.

Other ways in which drugs can act on cell processes is by acting on enzymes which can promote or accelerate biochemical reactions, and the action of a drug depends upon the role of the enzyme it affects. An example is angiotensin converting enzyme (ACE) which converts angiotensin I to II (which is a potent vasoconstrictor) increasing blood pressure. ACE inhibitors – as their name implies – prevent this conversion reducing blood pressure. An example is lisinopril.

Ion channels

Some systems are controlled by movement of certain ions (through channels known as ion channels) in and out of cells. Drugs can block these channels, which interferes with ion transport and therefore causes an altered response.

An example is the movement of calcium ions in constriction of blood vessels. Calcium channels open allowing calcium ions to pass into muscle cells of blood vessels causing them to constrict. This in turn reduces the diameter of the blood vessels which increases blood pressure. Calcium channel blockers such as nifedipine act by occupying these calcium channels and preventing the calcium ions passing through and exerting their effect. This means that the muscle cells cannot contract but relax, causing a lowering of blood pressure.

Carrier or transport mechanisms

These are energy-dependent transport systems, and some drugs can interfere with these mechanisms by acting as carrier inhibitors.

Examples include digoxin, which blocks the sodium pump in the heart, and omeprazole, which blocks the potassium pump in the gastric mucosa.

Others
Cancer drugs act by interfering with cell growth and division. Antibiotics act by interfering with the cell processes of invading bacteria and other micro-organisms.

References

Hopkins SJ. *Drugs and Pharmacology for Nurses* (1999). 13th ed. Churchill-Livingstone, Edinburgh.

Grahame-Smith DG, Aronson JK. *Oxford Textbook of Clinical Pharmacology and Drug Therapy* (2002). 3rd ed. Oxford University Press, Oxford.

Drug Safety Update, 6(12); July 2013: A1. Medicines and Healthcare Products Regulatory Agency (MHRA). http://www.mhra.gov.uk/. Accessed February 5, 2014: http://www.mhra.gov.uk/home/groups/dsu/documents/publication/con296410.pdf

ADMINISTRATION OF MEDICINES

There are several routes of administration. The route of administration depends upon:

- Which is the most convenient route for the patient
- The drug and its properties
- The formulations available
- How quick an effect is required
- Whether a local or systemic effect is required
- The clinical condition of the patient – the oral route may not be possible
- Whether the patient is compliant or not

We will look at two of the most common routes of administration, oral and parenteral.

Oral administration

For most patients, the oral route is the most convenient and acceptable way for taking medicines. Drugs may be given as tablets, capsules or liquids; other means include orodispersible, buccal or sublingual administration.

Advantages
- Convenient and allows self-administration
- Cheap; there is no need for special equipment

- Avoids fear of needles
- The GI tract provides a large surface area for absorption

Disadvantages
- Not all drugs activate orally
- Must be swallowed which may not always be possible
- Delayed onset of action due to the fact that drugs must be absorbed before they can act
- Absorption can be variable due to:
  - The presence of food
  - Interactions
  - Gastric emptying
    - Undergoes 'first-pass' metabolism
    - Patient needs to remember to take doses
- Possible gastric adverse effects

Formulations
Apart from the active drug, tablets and capsules may contain other ingredients that are needed for their manufacture, stability, administration or absorption. Patients may be allergic to some of these ingredients, including:

- Lactose – filler
- Preservatives – for stability
- E-numbers – for colourings and flavourings
- Sucrose – for flavouring, and can act as a binder

As a nurse, it is important to know the allergy status of a patient before administering or prescribing a medicine.

Enteric-coated (EC) preparations have a coating that prevents dissolution in the acid environment of the stomach, but acts to dissolve them in the intestines. The purpose is to:

- Protect the stomach from irritant drugs (can cause stomach ulcers)
- Prevent the stomach acid affecting the drug
- Allow release at the intended site, i.e. in the intestines

Modified release (can be designated as MR, SR, CR, XL or LA) preparations are designed to slowly release drugs (over 12 to 24 hours) to reduce the need of repeated dosing for drugs with short half-lives.

It is important for nurses to not crush tablets or open capsules that are modified release preparations. Patients must also be informed not to do the same, or to chew them.

As mentioned, a major disadvantage of the oral route is that drugs can undergo 'first-pass' metabolism; taking medicines by the sublingual or buccal route avoids this as the medicines enter directly into the bloodstream through the oral mucosa.

With sublingual administration the drug is put under the tongue where it dissolves in salivary secretions; with buccal administration the drug is placed between the gum and the mucous membrane of the cheek. Absorption can be rapid, so drug effects can be seen within a few minutes, e.g. sublingual GTN tablets. A problem with these two routes (particularly sublingual) is that a dry mouth may affect absorption. Don't forget – some drugs may cause dry mouth as a side effect.

Practical implications

Liquid medicines are usually measured with a 5 mL spoon. For other doses, oral syringes or medicine measures are used.

Medicine measures

These are used on the ward to measure individual patient doses. They measure volumes ranging from 5 to 30 mL and are not meant to be 100% accurate. The gradation mark to which you are measuring should be at eye level. If viewed from above, the level may appear higher than it really is; if viewed from below, it appears lower.

Oral syringes

These are useful for measuring doses less than 5 mL. Oral syringes are available in various sizes; an example is the Baxa Exacta-Med® range.

Oral syringe calibrations

You should use the most appropriate syringe for your dose, and calculate your answers for doses according to the syringe.

SYRINGE SIZE	GRADATIONS	ANSWER (ML)
0.5 mL, 1 mL	0.01 mL	Two decimal places
2 mL, 3 mL	0.1 mL	One decimal place
5 mL, 10 mL	0.2 mL	Round up or down to the nearest 0.2 mL multiple
20 mL, 35 mL, 60 mL	1 mL	Round up or down to the nearest mL

As with syringes for parenteral use, you should not try to administer the small amount of liquid that is left in the nozzle of the syringe after administering the drug. This small volume is known as 'dead space' or 'dead volume'. However, there are concerns with this 'dead space' when administering small doses and administering to babies. If dose volumes are small, the trapped fluid may represent a considerable proportion of the intended dose. In addition, if a baby is allowed to suck on an oral syringe, there is a danger that the baby will suck all of the medicine out of the syringe (including the amount contained in the 'dead space') and may inadvertently take too much.

A part of the design of an oral syringe is that it should not be possible to attach a needle to the nozzle. This prevents the accidental intravenous administration of an oral preparation. The problem was highlighted by the National Patient Safety Agency (NPSA) bulletin *Promoting Safer Measurement and Administration of Liquid Medicines via Oral and Other Enteral Routes* (March 2007); http://www.npsa.nhs.uk/nrls/alerts-and-directives/alerts/liquid-medicines/

Parenteral administration of drugs

This is the injection of drugs directly into the blood or tissues. The three most common methods are intravenous (IV), subcutaneous (SC) and intramuscular (IM).

Intravenous (IV) injection
The drug is injected directly into a vein, usually in the arm or hand.

Administering drugs by the IV route can be associated with problems, so a definite decision must be made to use the IV route and only if no other route is appropriate. Situations in which IV therapy would be appropriate are when:

- The patient is unable to take or tolerate oral medication, or has problems with absorption.
- High drug levels are needed rapidly which cannot be achieved by another route because they
  - are not absorbed orally,
  - are inactivated by the gut, or
  - undergo extensive first-pass metabolism.
- Constant drug levels are needed (such as those achieved by a continuous infusion).

Drugs have a very short elimination half-life $(t_{1/2})$. If you remember from the section on pharmacokinetics, the elimination half-life is the time taken for the concentration or level of a drug in the blood or plasma to fall to half its original value. Drugs with very short half-lives disappear from the bloodstream quickly and may need to be administered by a continuous infusion to maintain a clinical effect.

Advantages
- A rapid onset of action and response is achieved since it bypasses the gastrointestinal tract and first-pass metabolism.
- A constant and predictable therapeutic effect can be attained.

- IV administration can be used for drugs that are irritant or unpredictable when administered IM (e.g. patients with small muscle mass, who may have thrombocytopenia, or have haemophilia).
- The IV route allows for administration when the oral route cannot be used (e.g. when patients are nil-by-mouth, at risk of aspiration or suffering from nausea and vomiting).
- Drugs can be administered to patients who are unconscious.
- Fluid and electrolyte imbalances can be quickly corrected.

Disadvantages

- Training is required – not only on how to use the equipment, but also on calculating doses and rates of infusion.
- There is a high cost associated with IV administration:
  - Cost of pumps and giving sets
  - Cost of training
- There may be patient factors associated with IV administration:
  - Apprehension and fear associated with needles
  - Lack of mobility
- Several risks are associated with the IV route:
  - Toxicity – side effects usually more immediate and severe
  - Accidental overdose
  - Embolism
  - Microbial contamination/infection
  - Phlebitis/thrombophlebitis
  - Extravasation
  - Particulate contamination
  - Fluid overload
  - Compatibility/stability problems

Methods of intravenous administration

Intravenous bolus

This is the administration of a small volume (usually up to 10 mL) into a cannula or the injection site of an administration set – over 3 to 5 minutes unless otherwise specified.
Indications

- To achieve immediate and high drug levels – as in an emergency
- To ensure that medicines that are inactivated very rapidly, e.g. adenosine used to treat arrhythmias, produce a clinical effect
- May allow self-administration
- When the patient is fluid restricted
- When time is limited as with anaesthetics – it is not practical to wait a prolonged period of time for the anaesthetic to be administered

Drawbacks

- Only small volumes can be administered
- Tendency to administer the dose too rapidly which may be associated with increased adverse events for some medicines, e.g. vancomycin ('red man syndrome')
- Injection unlikely to be able to be stopped if an adverse event occurs
- Damage to the veins, e.g. phlebitis or extravasation, especially with potentially irritant medicines

Intermittent intravenous infusion

This is the administration of a small volume infusion (usually up to 250 mL) over a given time (usually 20 minutes to 2 hours), either as a one-off dose or repeated at specific time intervals. It is often a compromise between a bolus injection and continuous infusion in that it can achieve high plasma concentrations rapidly to ensure clinical efficacy and yet reduce the risk of adverse reactions associated with rapid administration.

Continuous intravenous infusion

This is the administration of a larger volume (usually between 500 mL and 3 litres) over a number of hours. Continuous infusions are usually used to replace fluids and to correct electrolyte imbalances. Sometimes drugs are added in order to produce a constant effect, e.g. as with analgesics – usually given as small-volume infusions (e.g. 50 mL) via syringe drivers.

Indications (intermittent infusions)

- When a drug must be diluted in a volume of fluid larger than is practical for a bolus injection
- When plasma levels need to be higher than those that can be achieved by continuous infusion
- When a faster response is required than that from a continuous infusion
- When a drug would be unstable when given as a continuous infusion

Indications (continuous infusions)

- When a constant therapeutic effect is required or to maintain adequate plasma concentrations
- When a medicine has a rapid elimination rate or short half-life and can have an effect only if given continuously

Drawbacks (both)

- Volume of diluent may cause fluid overload in susceptible patients (e.g. the elderly, those with heart or renal failure)
- Incompatibility problems with the infusion fluid
- Incomplete mixing of solutions
- Training is required – calculation skills for accurate determination of infusion concentration and rates; knowledge of, and competence in, operating infusion devices
- Increased risk of microbial and particulate contamination during preparation
- Risk of complications, such as haematomas, phlebitis, and extravasation

Subcutaneous (SC) injection

The SC route is generally used for administering small volumes (up to 2 mL) of nonirritant drugs such as insulin and heparin. Subcutaneous injections are usually given into the fatty layer directly below the skin; absorption is greater when compared with the oral route as the drug will be absorbed via the capillaries.

Advantages
- Patient can self-administer.
- First-pass metabolism is avoided.
- Slower or more prolonged plasma peak levels are possible than with the IV route.
- Large volume infusions are possible by the SC route over a prolonged period of time (usually over 24 hours) – a procedure known as hypodermoclysis.

Disadvantages
- Care must be taken not to inject IV.
- SC injection can produce some discomfort.
- Complications can arise, e.g. bruising.

Intramuscular (IM) injection

The IM route is generally used for the administration of drugs in the form of suspensions or oily solutions (usually no more than 3 mL). Absorption from IM injections can be variable and depends upon which muscle is used and the rate of perfusion through the muscle. (This can be increased by gently massaging the site of the injection.)

Advantages
- It is easier to give than an IV infusion.
- First-pass metabolism is avoided.

- Aqueous drugs are absorbed rapidly.
- A depot effect is possible – drugs dispersed in oil are absorbed more slowly.

Disadvantages
- Injection can be painful.
- Self-administration is difficult.
- Complications can arise, e.g. bruising or abscesses.
- Avoid in patients with clotting disorders.

Figure 10.7 shows plasma profiles of drugs administered via different routes.

Practical aspects
As with oral syringes, syringes for parenteral use are available in various sizes. Once again, you should use the most appropriate syringe for your dose, and calculate your answers for doses according to the syringe. For example:

SYRINGE SIZE	GRADATIONS	ANSWER (ML)
1 mL	0.01 mL	Two decimal places
2 mL	0.1 mL	One decimal place
5 mL	0.2 mL	Round up or down to the nearest 0.2 mL multiple
10 mL	0.5 mL	Round up or down to the nearest 0.5 mL multiple
20 mL, 30 mL, 50 mL	1 mL	Round up or down to the nearest mL

As with syringes for oral use, there is also a 'dead space' or 'dead volume' with an associated volume, which is taken into account

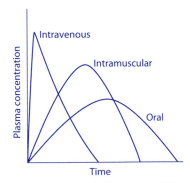

Figure 10.7 Plasma profiles of drugs administered via different routes.

by the manufacturer. When measuring volume with a syringe, it is important to expel all the air first before adjusting to the final volume. The volume is measured from the bottom of the plunger.

You should not try to administer the small amount of liquid left in the nozzle of the syringe after administering the drug. This small volume is known as 'dead space' or 'dead volume'. However, there are concerns with this 'dead space' when administering small doses and to babies, particularly if the dose is diluted before administration. For example, if a drug is drawn up to the 0.02 mL mark of a 1 mL syringe and injected directly, the drug in the dead space is retained in the syringe, and there is no overdose delivered. However, when a diluent is drawn up into the syringe for dilution, the drug in the dead space is also drawn up, and this results in possible overdosing.

PROMOTING THE SAFER USE OF INJECTABLE MEDICINES

The risks associated with using injectable medicines in clinical areas have been recognized and well known for some time. Evidence indicates that the incidence of errors in prescribing, preparing and administering injectable medicines is higher than for other forms of medicine. As a consequence the National Patient Safety Agency (NPSA) issued safety alert 20 – *Promoting Safer Use of Injectable Medicines* – in March 2007.

The NPSA highlighted eight risks associated with the prescribing, preparing and administering of injectable drugs.

Two risks which highlight the involvement of calculations and so emphasize the need to be able to perform calculations confidently and competently are shown in the following table.

	RISK FACTORS	DESCRIPTION
3	**Complex calculation**	Any calculation with more than one step required for preparation and/or administration, e.g. microgram/kg/hour, dose unit conversion such as mg to mmol or % to mg.
7	**Use of a pump or syringe driver**	All pumps and syringe drivers require some element of calculation and therefore have potential for error and should be included in the risk factors. However, it is important to note that this potential risk is considered less significant than the risks associated with not using a pump when indicated.

Hospitals must ensure that healthcare staff who prescribe, prepare and administer injectable medicines have received training and have the necessary work competences to undertake their duties safely. This includes IV study days which will teach nurses to be able to prepare and administer injectable drugs, and subsequently assess them on their knowledge. Some of these assessments will involve drug calculations.

Reference

http://www.npsa.nhs.uk/nrls/alerts-and-directives/alerts/injectable-
medicines/

PROBLEMS

Write down the volume as indicated for the following syringes:

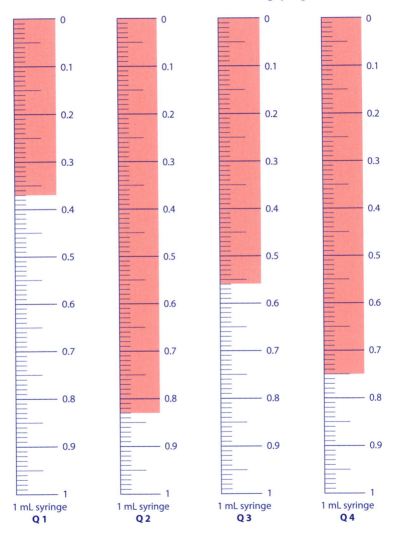

| 1 mL syringe | 1 mL syringe | 1 mL syringe | 1 mL syringe |
| **Q 1** | **Q 2** | **Q 3** | **Q 4** |

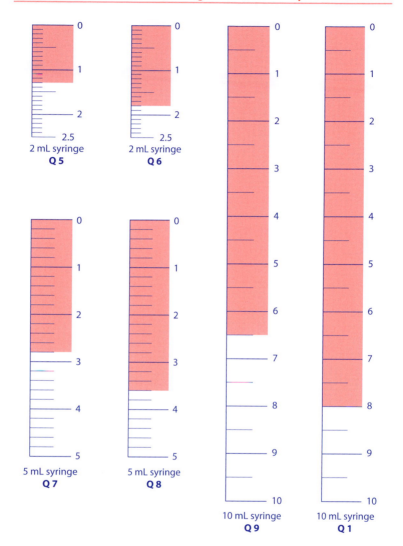

2 mL syringe
Q 5

2 mL syringe
Q 6

5 mL syringe
Q 7

5 mL syringe
Q 8

10 mL syringe
Q 9

10 mL syringe
Q 1

Answers can be found in Chapter 15.

11 CHILDREN AND MEDICINES

OBJECTIVES

At the end of this chapter, you should be familiar with the following:

- Drug handling in children
- Routes of administration
  - Oral administration
  - Parenteral administration
- Practical implications
  - General
  - Dosing
  - Licensing and 'off-label' use
  - Formulations
  - Problems associated with paediatric doses
- Useful reference books
- Approximate values useful in the calculation of doses in children
- Calculating dosages

KEY POINTS

Prescribing in paediatrics

- Doses are usually prescribed on a weight (mg/kg) or surface area (mg/m^2) basis; the use of formulae is no longer recommended.

Drug handling and drug response

- Drug handling (pharmacokinetcs) and drug response (pharmacodynamics) may change, particularly in neonates.
- Doses of some drugs may have to be increased or reduced depending on how they are absorbed, broken down or metabolized, distributed or excreted.

Routes of administration

- These are largely determined mainly by the age and how ill the child is.
- In the sick premature newborn, almost all drugs are given IV.
- In full-term newborns, and older children, the oral route is the easiest and most convenient route, particularly for long-term treatment. However, for the acutely ill child and for children with vomiting, diarrhoea and impaired GI function, the parenteral route is recommended.

Practical implications

- If possible, children should know why they need a medicine and be shown how they can take it.

- Young children and infants who cannot understand will usually take medicine from someone they know and trust – a parent or main carer. So, it is important that those who give medicines know about the medicine and how to give it.
- Occasionally, there may be problems in giving medicines – usually due to taste, swallowing a tablet or capsule, or strengths of medicines available. In these cases a liquid preparation is necessary – either available commercially or specially made.
- Some medicines, particularly commercially available ones, may contain excipients (e.g. alcohol) which may cause problems in children – prescribers and those administering medicines should take this into account.

INTRODUCTION

The *National Service Framework (NSF) – Medicines for Children and Young People* (DH 2004) states: 'Children, young people, their parents or carers, and healthcare professionals in all settings make decisions about medicines based on sound information about risk and benefit. They have access to safe and effective medicines that are prescribed on the basis of the best available evidence.'

The aims of the framework are to ensure that all children and young people:

- receive medicines that are safe and effective, in formulations that can easily be administered and are appropriate to their age, having minimum impact on their education and lifestyle.
- are cared for by professionals who are well-trained, informed, and competent to work with children to improve health outcomes and minimize harm and any side effects of medicines.
- are (along with their parents or carers) well-informed and supported to make choices about their medicines and are competent in the administration of medicines.

Children are very different from adults and shouldn't be considered as small adults when prescribing medicines. This is certainly true for how children handle and respond to drugs. An understanding of the likely changes that can occur as children grow is important for the administration of medicines – and also for an awareness of when children can swallow tablets, open bottles, read information and so on.

As knowledge has increased, the use of formulae to estimate children's doses based on those of adults is no longer recommended. Doses are given either in terms of body weight (mg/kg) or body surface area (mg/m^2) in an attempt to take developmental changes into account.

Table 11.1 Age ranges and definitions

DEFINITION	AGE RANGE
Preterm newborn infants	<37 weeks' gestation
Term newborn infants	0–27 days
Infants and toddlers	28 days–23 months
Children	2–11 years
Adolescents	12–16 or 18 years

Note: These age ranges are intended to reflect biological changes.

The International Committee on Harmonization (2000) has suggested that childhood be divided into the age ranges shown in Table 11.1 for the purposes of clinical trials and licensing of medicines.

Reference

Department of Health (DH). *The National Service Framework (NSF) – Medicines for Children and Young People*. London, October 2004.

DRUG HANDLING IN CHILDREN

As noted earlier, children are different from adults in the way that they handle and respond to drugs. Age-related differences in drug handling (pharmacokinetics) and drug sensitivity (pharmacodynamics) occur throughout childhood and account for many of the differences between drug doses at various stages of childhood. Many drugs used in paediatrics have not been studied adequately or at all in children, so prescribing for children may not always be easy.

Drug absorption

There are various differences between children and adults which can affect the way in which drugs are absorbed orally. Changes in the gastric acid production, gastric emptying or motility, and intestinal enzymes are the main factors on the rate and extent of oral absorption. In neonates, there is reduced gastric acid secretion; at 2 years, acid production increases and is comparable to adults. Gastric motility reaches normality at about 6 months of age.

There is some evidence to suggest that in neonates and young infants, up to the age of 4–6 months, the rate of absorption is slower and the time taken to reach maximum blood levels is therefore longer. Vomiting or acute diarrhoea, which is particularly common during childhood, may dramatically reduce the extent of drug absorption by reducing the time that the drug remains in the small intestine. This means that drugs may have a reduced effect and therefore may have to be given by another route.

Other factors affecting absorption include the immature biliary system, which may affect the absorption and transport of fat-soluble (lipophilic) drugs. In addition, the activity of drug-metabolizing enzymes in the liver and bacterial microflora in the gut may vary with age, and this may lead to different and unpredictable oral drug absorption in neonates and young infants.

Because the absorption of oral drugs is unpredictable in neonates, the oral route is not really used to treat acute conditions. However, once the neonate is taking full feeds, oral absorption may be more predictable.

Drug distribution

Factors that affect drug distribution vary with age. The distribution of a drug to its site of action influences its therapeutic and adverse effects. This may vary considerably in neonates and young infants resulting in a different therapeutic or adverse effect from that which is expected.

In general, changes in body composition (body water and fat) can alter the way that drugs are distributed round the body. The most dramatic changes occur in the first year of life but continue throughout puberty and adolescence, particularly the proportion of total body fat. The extent to which a drug distributes between fat and water depends upon its physiochemical properties, i.e. according to how they dissolve in water (water solubility) and in fat (lipid solubility). Water-soluble drugs are mainly distributed within the extracellular space and fat-soluble drugs within fat.

Neonates and infants have relatively large extracellular fluid and total body water spaces compared with adults, resulting in a larger apparent volume of distribution of drugs that distribute into these spaces and lower plasma concentrations for the same weight-based dose, and so higher doses of water-soluble drugs are required.

Another major determinant of drug distribution is protein binding. A certain proportion of drug will be bound to plasma proteins and a proportion will be unbound – only the unbound drug is able to go to its site of action. Protein binding is reduced in neonates due to reduced albumin and plasma protein concentrations, but increases with age and reaches adult levels by about one year.

For drugs that are highly protein bound, small changes in the binding of the drug can make a large difference to the free drug concentration if the drug is displaced. As a consequence, lower total plasma concentrations of some drugs may be required to achieve a therapeutic effect. Drugs affected include phenytoin, phenobarbital and furosemide.

This change in binding is also important with regard to bilirubin in neonates. Bilirubin is a breakdown product of old blood cells that is carried in the blood (by binding to plasma proteins) to the liver where it is chemically modified (by conjugation) and then excreted in the bile into the newborn's digestive tract. Displacement by drugs and the immature conjugating mechanisms of the liver means that unconjugated bilirubin levels can rise and can cross the brain–blood barrier. High levels cause kernicterus (brain damage). Conversely, high circulating bilirubin levels in neonates may displace drugs from proteins.

Metabolism

The primary organ for drug breakdown or metabolism is the liver. In the first weeks of life, the ability of the liver to metabolize drugs is not fully developed and the different systems mature at different times. This all changes in the 1–9 age group, and the metabolic clearance of drugs is shown to be greater than in adults – probably due to the relatively large size of the liver compared to body size and maturation of the enzyme systems. Thus to achieve plasma concentrations similar to those seen in adults, dosing in this group may need to be higher.

Elimination

In neonates, the immaturity of the kidney, particularly glomerular filtration and active tubular secretion and reabsorption of drugs, limits the ability to renally excrete drugs. Below 3–6 months of age, glomerular filtration is less than that of adults, but may be partially compensated by a relatively greater reduction in tubular reabsorption as tubular function matures at a slower rate. However, drugs may accumulate leading to toxic effects. Maturity of renal function occurs toward 6–8 months of age. After 8–12 months, function is similar to that seen in older children and adults.

PHARMACODYNAMICS

There is little known about how drugs interact with receptors in children, but there may be age differences for certain drugs, e.g. digoxin, warfarin.

ROUTES OF ADMINISTRATION OF DRUGS

These are determined mainly by the age and how ill the child is. In the sick premature newborn, almost all drugs are given IV since GI function and therefore drug absorption are impaired. (IM is not suitable as there is very poor muscle mass.)

In full-term newborns and older children, the oral route is the easiest and most convenient one, particularly for long-term treatment. However, for the acutely ill child and for children with vomiting, diarrhoea and impaired GI function, the parenteral route is recommended.

Oral administration

It is not always possible to give tablets or capsules: either the dose required does not exist, or the child cannot swallow tablets or capsules (children under 5 years are unlikely to accept tablets or capsules). Therefore an oral liquid preparation is necessary, either as a ready-made preparation or one made especially by the pharmacy. Older children also often prefer liquids. Liquid formulations sometimes have the disadvantage of an unpleasant taste and this may be disguised by flavouring or by mixing them with, or following them immediately by, favourite foods or drinks. However, mixing the drugs with food may cause dosage problems and affect absorption. It is worth remembering that to ensure adequate dosing, all of the medicine and food must be taken.

Parents and carers should be discouraged from adding medicines to a baby's bottle. This is because of potential interactions with milk feeds and under dosing if not all the feed is taken. The crushing or opening of slow-release tablets and capsules should also be discouraged; this should only be done on advice from pharmacy.

Domestic teaspoons vary in size and are not a reliable measure. A 5 mL medicine spoon or an oral syringe should be used, and parents or carers may need to be shown how to use these (see the section on oral syringes in Chapter 10).

Parenteral administration

The parenteral route is the most reliable with regard to obtaining predictable blood levels; giving drugs intravenously is the most commonly used parenteral route. It is now commonplace to use infusion pumps when giving infusions rather than using a paediatric or micro-drop giving set on its own, as pumps are considered to be more accurate and safer.

Intramuscular (IM)

Although most drugs can be injected into muscle, the IM route should be avoided if at all possible. This is because of:

- Reduced muscle mass
- Reduced muscle blood flow
- Low concentrations of drug achieved
- Unpredictable dosing due to the pain it causes

In practice, the route is used for concentrated and irritating solutions which may cause local pain if injected subcutaneously and which cannot be given by any other way.

In a child who has already received several days of intravenous antibiotics and in whom cannulation has become difficult, two or three days of a once-a-day IM injection to complete the course may be preferable to multiple intravenous cannulation attempts which may cause stress and distress to the child. Thin infants may be given 1–2 mL and bigger children 1–5 mL, using needles of appropriate length for the site chosen. The shorter and the narrower the needle, the less pain it will cause.

Intravenous (IV)

In hospital practice, drugs not given orally are usually given IV rather than SC or IM, as the effect is quicker and more predictable, the pain of multiple injections is avoided, and larger volumes can be given. However, in neonates, due to the fragility of the veins, extravasation is relatively common and can cause problems if drugs leak into the tissues. Central venous access is used for children who need irritant or cardiac drugs, administration of medicines over long periods, and for home therapy with IV drugs.

Other routes of administration

- *Rectal* – absorption in neonates may be slow and unpredictable, although it is a useful option when other routes are unavailable.
- *Buccal* – this is a useful option for certain drugs, e.g. midazolam for the acute treatment of seizures instead of rectal diazepam.

PRACTICAL IMPLICATIONS

General

In the United Kingdom, the *British National Formulary for Children* (BNF-C) (see *Further Reading* section) is a national formulary which includes prescribing guidelines and drug monographs. You should read the relevant sections.

If possible, children should know why they need a medicine and be shown how they can take it. Young children and infants who cannot understand will usually take medicine from someone they know and trust – a parent or main carer. Therefore it is important that those who give medicines know about the medicine and how to give it. Occasionally, there may be problems in giving medicines – usually due to taste or difficulty swallowing a tablet or capsule. Parents or carers should not give in to fractious children and should not give medicines, as then compliance may be a problem; at all stages, the child should be comforted and reassured. The child must not be left with the impression that being given medicine is a punishment for being sick.

Another problem is that the child may seem better so parents/carers may not complete treatment, as in antibiotics. The approach depends on the child's understanding and the circumstances:

- *Under 2 years*. Administration by parents if possible, using an approach which they believe is most likely to succeed.
- *2 to 5 year olds* need a calm, gentle, firm, and efficient approach after they have been told what is happening. Play and acting out may help them understand. Rewards may encourage further co-operation.
- *5 to 12 year olds* also need encouragement, respect for their trust, and an explanation attuned to their understanding.
- *Over 12 years*. At this age children must have a proper understanding of what is happening and share in the decision making as well as the responsibility. They must feel in control.

What children and carers need to know
- The name of the medicine
- The reason for using it
- When and how to take it
- How to know if it is effective, and what to do if it is not
- What to do if one or more doses are missed
- How long to continue taking it
- The risks of stopping it
- The most likely adverse effects; those unlikely, but important; and what to do if they occur
- Whether other medicines can be taken at the same time
- Whether other remedies alter the medicine's effect

Nursing staff involved with children need to remember about medicines and dosage problems in children.

Dosing

Most doses of medicines have been derived from trials or from clinical experience, and the nature of the drug should decide as to which method of dose calculation is the most appropriate. Drugs with a critical, narrow therapeutic index (i.e. a small difference between the effective and toxic dose), such as cytotoxics, require an accurate method – dosing based on body surface area. Using body surface area may be the most accurate method for dosing, as surface area better reflects developmental changes and function. However, the downside to this method is that it is not always easy, and it is time consuming to obtain accurate measurements for height and weight; so this is generally reserved for the potent drugs where there are small differences between effective and toxic doses.

Drugs with a wide therapeutic index (i.e. a large difference between the effective and toxic dose), such as penicillins, allow for some flexibility in dosing so an approximation is suitable – dosing based on a given dose or on a weight basis. A dose solely based on a weight basis (mg/kg) assumes that the dose is appropriate for a particular child or age. However, this may not be correct due to a variety of factors such as disease, prematurity or obesity. Also, remember that children grow at different rates, so a 'one size fits all' approach does not always apply. Before a dose is prescribed/given, appropriateness of the child's weight and height should be re-assessed. Both methods rely on accurate weight and height measurements. Most drugs have a wide safety margin, so an alternative method of dosing is by age banding, and this is a much easier way of dosing. For example: paracetamol, the BNF for Children (2014–15) gives the following:

Oral paracetamol

CHILD AGE RANGE	DOSE	MAX DOSES/HR
1–3 months	30–60 mg every 8 hr as necessary	60 mg/kg daily in divided doses
3–6 months	60 mg every 4–6 hr	4 doses/24 hr
6 months–2 years	120 mg every 4–6 hr	4 doses/24 hr
2–4 years	180 mg every 4–6 hr	4 doses/24 hr
4–6 years	240 mg every 4–6 hr	4 doses/24 hr
6–8 years	240–250 mg every 4–6 hr	4 doses/24 hr
8–10 years	360–375 mg every 4–6 hr	4 doses/24 hr
10–12 years	480–500 mg every 4–6 hr	4 doses/24 hr
12–16 years	480–750 mg every 4–6 hr	4 doses/24 hr
16–18 years	500 mg–1 g every 4–6 hr	4 doses/24 hr

Once again, the appropriateness of the dose for the individual child, who may be small or large for their age, should always be assessed.

MAKE SURE THAT PAEDIATRIC
DOSES ARE CHECKED CAREFULLY

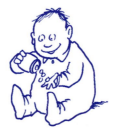

Licensing and 'off-label' use

Many drugs are not tested in children, which means that they are not specifically licensed for use in children. So although a medicine may be licensed, it may often be prescribed outside the terms of its Marketing Authorisation (or licence) – known as 'off-label' prescribing – in relation to age, indication, dose of frequency, route of administration or formulation. Using medicines that are not licensed means that there is limited information on safety, quality and efficacy, and a potentially increased risk of side effects or adverse drug reactions.

The Joint Royal College of Paediatrics and Child Health and the Neonatal and Paediatric Pharmacists Group (RCPH/NPPG) Standing Committee on Medicines issued a policy statement (2000, updated 2013):

- Those who prescribe for a child should choose the medicine which offers the best prospect for that child, aware that such prescribing may be constrained by the availability of resources. Children should be able to receive medicines that are safe, effective, appropriate for their condition, palatable and available with minimal clinical risk.
- The informed use of some unlicensed medicines or licensed medicines for unlicensed applications is necessary in paediatric practice.
- Health professionals should have access to reliable and up-to-date information where possible on any medicine they prescribe, dispense or administer, and on its availability.
- In general, it is not necessary to take additional steps beyond those taken when prescribing licensed medicines to obtain the consent of parents, carers and child patients to prescribe or administer unlicensed medicines or licensed medicines for unlicensed applications.
- NHS Trusts and Health Authorities should support therapeutic practices that are advocated by a respectable, responsible body of professional opinion.
- Where available, an appropriate licensed preparation should be prescribed and supplied in preference to an unlicensed preparation.

Nursing staff should be aware when an unlicensed medicine is being administered as well as aware of their responsibilities.

Formulations

Appropriate formulations to enable administration of drugs to children are often not available. Children may not be able to swallow tablets or capsules, so liquid medicines are preferred. However, this is not always available and crushing of tablets or manipulation of solid dosage forms into suspensions or powders is often required. Be aware that this is an unlicensed method of administration, not all of the prescribed dose may be given, and there may be safety issues – inhalation or skin sensitization problems may occur. Always seek advice from pharmacy before doing or advising this.

Even parenteral medicines are only available in adult dose sizes. The strength of these products may mean that it is difficult to measure small doses for children and may lead to errors. Some commercially available medicines may contain excipients that could cause adverse effects or be inappropriate to use in some children. Liquid preparations may contain excipients such as alcohol, sorbitol, propylene glycol or E-numbers; sugar-free medicines should be dispensed whenever possible. Parenteral products may contain benzyl alcohol or propylene glycol which also can cause adverse effects such as metabolic acidosis.

Problems associated with paediatric dosing

In addition to changes in how the body handles drugs, doses may have to be adjusted for fever, oedema, dehydration and GI disease. In these cases, the doctor should decide whether a dose needs to be adjusted.

There will also be occasions when it is difficult to give the dose required due to the lack of an appropriate formulation; for example, to give 33 mg when only a 100 mg tablet is available. In these instances, it is advisable that the pharmacy department be contacted to see if a liquid preparation is available or can be prepared. If not, the doctor should be informed so that the dose can be modified, another drug can be prescribed or another route can be used.

Another problem is frequency of dosing; with children, particularly young children, the waking day is much shorter compared to that of adults. A drug prescribed to be given four times a day may not be practical to be given in a short waking period. In addition, dosing during the day will mean doses may have to be given at school which may not always be easy or possible. Medicines may have to be changed to ones that can be given once or twice daily outside school hours. The ideal medicine for a child should have the following attributes:

- Dosing to suit all age groups
- Minimal dosage frequency
- Palatability
- Contain few, nontoxic excipients
- Be easy for the child to take or for the carer to administer
- Have a stable formulation
- Be commercially viable

Unfortunately, this is not always possible, and healthcare professionals involved in prescribing, supplying and administering medicines should be aware of the potential problems and should assess each individual child and their circumstances to ensure that the child gains the most benefit from the medicines, especially in chronic, long-term conditions.

References

Anon. *Medicines for Children 2003* (2003) 2nd ed. Royal College of Paediatrics and Child Health and Neonatal and Paediatric Pharmacists Group. RCPCH Publications, London.

British National Formulary for Children 2014–15 (2014). Pharmaceutical Press, London.

Costello I, Long PF, Wong IK, Tuleu C, Yeung V. *Paediatric Drug Handling* (2007). Pharmaceutical Press, London.

Grahame-Smith DG, Aronson JK. *Oxford Textbook of Clinical Pharmacology and Drug Therapy* (2001). 3rd ed. Oxford University Press, Oxford.

The Joint Royal College of Paediatrics and Child Health and the Neonatal and Paediatric Pharmacists Group (RCPH/NPPG) Standing Committee on Medicines. *The Use of Unlicensed Medicines or Licensed Medicines for Unlicensed Applications in Paediatric Practice*, December 2013 (http://www.rcpch.ac.uk/child-health/childrens-medicines/childrens-medicines, accessed May 14, 2014).

Walker R, Whittlesea C (editors). *Clinical Pharmacy and Therapeutics* (2012). 5th ed. Churchill Livingstone, Oxford.

USEFUL REFERENCE BOOKS

Neonatal Formulary: Drug Use in Pregnancy and the First Year of Life – current edition (7th ed., 2014). Northern Neonatal Network, Wiley-Blackwell. Updates are available from: http://www.neonatalformulary.com

British National Formulary for Children (BNF-C) – current edition (latest edition, 2014–2015). Pharmaceutical Press, London. Also available online at http://www.medicinescomplete.com/mc/bnfc/current, http://www.bnf.org/bnf/index.htm *or* as a smartphone app via the NICE Website at http://www.nice.org.uk/aboutnice/nicewebsitedevelopment/NICEApps.jsp

APPROXIMATE VALUES USEFUL IN THE CALCULATION OF DOSES IN CHILDREN

The following table gives average values for various parameters. However, the child's actual weight and height might vary considerably from the values in the table, and it is important to see the child to ensure that the value chosen is appropriate. In most cases the child's actual measurement should be obtained as soon as possible and the dose recalculated.

AGE	WEIGHT (KG)	HEIGHT (CM)
Full-term neonate	3.5	51
1 month	4.3	55
2 months	5.4	58
3 months	6.1	61
4 months	6.7	63
6 months	7.6	67
1 year	9	75
3 years	14	96
5 years	18	109
7 years	23	122
10 years	32	138
12 years	39	149
14-year-old boy	49	163
14-year-old girl	50	159
Adult male	68	176
Adult female	58	164

Source: *British National Formulary for Children 2014–2015.* Pharmaceutical Press, London, 2014.

When doing any calculation, make sure that the decimal point is in the right place. A change to the left or right could mean a 10-fold change in the dose, which could be fatal in some cases.

It is best to work in the smaller units, i.e. 100 micrograms as opposed to 0.1 milligrams. Even so, care must be taken with the number of noughts; a wrong dose can be fatal.

When calculating any dose – always get your answer checked.

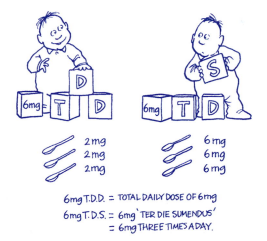

6mg T.D.D. = TOTAL DAILY DOSE OF 6mg
6mg T.D.S. = 6mg 'TER DIE SUMENDUS'
= 6mg THREE TIMES A DAY.

OBJECTIVES

At the end of this chapter, you should be familiar with the following:

- The elderly and medicines
- Drug handling in the elderly
- Specific problems in the elderly
- General principles

KEY POINTS

Prescribing in the elderly

- As a person grows older, it is inevitable that he or she will need some drug treatment.
- Changes in drug handling and response will occur.
- The elderly are more prone to adverse effects.
- The elderly have more compliance issues.

Drug handling and drug response

- Drug handling (pharmacokinetics) and drug response (pharmacodynamics) may change.
- Doses of some drugs may have to be reduced depending upon how they are absorbed, metabolized, distributed or excreted.

General principles

- Take a full medication history (including over-the-counter drugs).
- Choose the most suitable drug for the patient, considering:
  - the formulation
  - the frequency of administration (once versus four times a day)
  - the dose that may be necessary (start at a low dose and titrate slowly)
  - the disease and contraindications
- Keep the regime simple – use as few drugs as possible.
- Give clear and simple instructions.
- Establish that the patient can use the various compliance aids that are available.
- Consider the risk of drug interactions and adverse effects.
- Review medication regularly – do not continue to use a drug for longer than necessary.

INTRODUCTION

The 65 and over population in the United Kingdom is growing. Over the period 1985 to 2012 the number of people aged 65 and over in the United Kingdom increased by 26 per cent to 10.8 million; in 2012, 17 per cent of the population were aged 65 and over. The number of people aged 85 and over more than doubled over the same period to 1.4 million (Office for National Statistics 2014).

Population ageing will increase significantly for the next few decades. By 2037 the number of people aged 85 and over is projected to be 2.5 times larger than in 2012, reaching 3.6 million and accounting for 5 per cent of the total population. The population aged 65 and over will account for 24 per cent of the total population in 2037 (Office for National Statistics 2014).

As a person grows older, it is inevitable that some type(s) of drug treatment will be needed. Part of the ageing process is that physiological changes occur that affect how the elderly person handles and responds to drugs. The risk of adverse effects and drug interactions is also increased.

The National Service Framework (NSF) – Medicines and Older People (DH 2001) states that older people 'should have ready access to the right medicine, at the right dose and in the right form'. The aims of the Framework are to ensure that older people:

- Gain the maximum benefit from their medication to maintain or increase their quality and duration of life.
- Do not suffer unnecessarily from illness caused by excessive, inappropriate or inadequate consumption of medicines.

As people get older, their use of medicines tends to increase. Four in five people over 75 years take at least one prescribed medicine, with 36% taking four or five medicines (DH 2001).

DRUG HANDLING IN THE ELDERLY

Pharmacokinetics

Age-related changes in drug handling make older people more susceptible to drug effects.

Absorption

Changes in the gastrointestinal tract include a reduction in gastric acid output, reduction in surface area (due to atrophy of the mucosa), reduced blood flow, delay in gastric emptying, and decrease in active transport systems. Although there are numerous changes, the overall effect is not to change the extent of absorption, but to reduce the rate of absorption making it longer for a drug to have an effect and reach peak levels. For example, the absorption of some drugs such as digoxin may be slower, but the overall absorption is similar to that in the young.

Distribution

In older people, total body mass, lean body mass, and total body water decrease but total body fat increases. The effect of these changes on drug distribution depends on whether a drug is lipid or water soluble. A water-soluble drug is distributed mainly in the body water and lean body tissue. Because the elderly have relatively less water and lean tissue, more of a water-soluble drug stays in the blood, which leads to increased blood concentration levels. As a result, a reduction in dose may be required. Examples include digoxin and gentamicin.

As the elderly have a higher proportion of body fat, more of a fat-soluble drug is distributed in the body fat. This can produce misleadingly low blood levels and may cause dosage to be incorrectly increased. The fatty tissue slowly releases stored drug into the bloodstream, and this explains why a fat-soluble sedative may produce a hangover effect. Examples include diazepam and lidocaine. A decrease in albumin results in a reduction in the plasma protein binding of some drugs (e.g. phenytoin, warfarin). More non-bound drug is available to act at receptor sites and may result in toxicity. In these cases, a dose reduction may be necessary.

Metabolism

Metabolism deteriorates with age as blood flow to the liver deceases by about 40%, resulting in a reduction in first-pass metabolism. In addition, there is a decrease in liver size and enzyme synthesis, reducing the capacity of the liver to metabolize drugs. Metabolism may be further reduced by liver disease or dysfunction, which is more likely in the elderly. The result of all this may be increased blood levels and longer half-lives. Examples include NSAIDs, antiepileptics and analgesics. The nutritional status of a person can also have a marked influence on the rate of drug metabolism. In frail elderly patients, drug metabolism can be reduced to a greater extent than in the elderly with normal body weight.

Renal excretion

The most important and predictable pharmacokinetic change seen in the elderly is a reduction in renal drug clearance. As seen with the liver, various changes mean a reduction in the excretion of drugs. Changes include a reduction in kidney size, reduction in functioning nephrons, reduced blood flow with reduced glomerular filtration rate, and tubular secretion. A drug may accumulate (resulting in higher blood levels) if doses are not adjusted to account for the reduction in excretion by the kidneys. This decline in renal function can lead to an increase in adverse drug reactions, as the glomerular filtration rate can decrease to around 50 mL/min by the age of 80, so it is easier to predict adverse drug effects.

Drugs or active metabolites of those that are excreted mainly in the urine will require that the drug be given at lower doses, particularly those with a narrow therapeutic index (e.g. warfarin, digoxin, lithium, phenytoin and carbamazepine). Tetracyclines are best avoided in the elderly because they can accumulate, causing nausea and vomiting, and resulting in dehydration and further deterioration in renal function.

Disease states such as diabetes and heart failure can worsen renal function, as can an acute illness such as a chest infection that leads to dehydration.

Pharmacodynamics

The elderly appear to exhibit altered responses to drugs; in general, they have an increased sensitivity to drugs. This is due to probable changes in biomechanical responses, receptors, homeostatic changes and altered central nervous system (CNS) functions.

Homeostatic changes include orthostatic circulatory responses, postural control, thermoregulation and cognitive function. Orthostatic blood pressure control that prevents any fall in blood pressure, particularly when getting up quickly, may be impaired.

Along with postural hypotension, the elderly are more likely to suffer from drug-induced hypotension, which can lead to dizziness and falls. The thermoregulatory mechanisms are impaired, which may lead to some degree of hypothermia, particularly drug-induced hypothermia. This includes drugs that produce sedation, impaired subjective awareness of temperature, decreased mobility and muscular activity, and vasodilation. Commonly implicated drugs include phenothiazines, benzodiazepines, tricyclic antidepressants, opioids and alcohol, either on its own or with other drugs.

Cognitive function is affected by changes in the CNS which may be significant – movement disorders may be due to neurotransmitter changes and increased confusion due to reduced cerebral blood flow. The brain shows increased sensitivity to certain drugs, e.g. benzodiazepines, opioids, antiparkinsonian drugs and antidepressants – even at normal doses – with the result of patients becoming disorientated and confused.

There are changes in specific receptors and target sites – ageing can cause a reduction in number of receptors, and how receptors interact with drugs and cells. Examples include salbutamol (agonist) and propranolol (antagonist) – both will show a reduced effect.

SPECIFIC PROBLEMS IN THE ELDERLY

Constipation

Constipation is a common problem in the elderly due to a decline in gastrointestinal motility as a result of ageing. Anticholinergic drugs, opiates, tricyclic antidepressants and antihistamines are more likely to cause constipation in the elderly.

Urological problems

Anticholinergic drugs may cause urinary retention in elderly men, especially those who have prostatic hypertrophy. Bladder instability is common in the elderly, and urethral dysfunction is more prevalent in elderly women. Loop diuretics may cause incontinence in such patients.

Drug reactions

Psychotropic drugs

Hypnotics with long half-lives are a significant problem and can cause daytime drowsiness, unsteadiness from impaired balance, and confusion. Short-acting ones may also be a problem and should only be used for short periods if essential.

The elderly are more sensitive to benzodiazepines than the young, and the mechanism of this increased sensitivity is not known – smaller doses should be used. Tricyclic antidepressants can cause postural hypotension and confusion in the elderly.

Warfarin

The elderly are more sensitive to warfarin; doses can be about 25% less than in younger people. This phenomenon may be due to age-related changes in pharmacodynamic factors. The exact mechanism is unknown.

Digoxin

The elderly appear to be more sensitive to the adverse effects of digoxin, but not to the cardiac effects. Factors include potassium loss (which increases cell sensitivity to digoxin) due to diuretics and reduced renal excretion.

Diuretics

The elderly can easily lose too much fluid and become dehydrated, and this can affect treatment of hypotension. Diuretics can also cause extra potassium loss (hypokalaemia) which may increase the effects of digoxin and hence contribute to digoxin toxicity. The elderly can be more prone to gout because of the effect of diuretics causing uric acid retention (hyperuricaemia).

Compliance

Compliance can be a problem in the elderly, as complicated drug regimes may be difficult for them to follow so they either stop taking the drugs or take wrong doses at the wrong times. Dispensing drugs for elderly and confused people can be made easier by using various compliance aids. These are devices in which medication is dispensed for patients who experience difficulty in taking their medicines, particularly those who have difficulty in co-ordinating their medication regime or have a large number of medicines to take. Containers with compartments for each day of the week, with each compartment divided into four sections (i.e. morning, lunch, dinner, bedtime) are available. These do not benefit all types of patients and are not useful for patients who have visual impairment, dexterity problems or severe cognitive impairment.

Adverse reactions

An adverse reaction to a drug is likely to be two or three times more common in the elderly than in other patients. Some reasons for this are the following:

- Elderly patients often need several drugs at the same time, and there is a close relationship between the number of drugs taken and the incidence of adverse reactions.
- Pharmacokinetics in the elderly (how they handle drugs) may be impaired so that they may experience higher concentrations of some drugs unless the dose is suitably adjusted.
- Drugs associated with adverse reactions such as digoxin, diuretics, NSAIDs, hypotensives and various centrally acting agents are often prescribed for elderly patients.

GENERAL PRINCIPLES

Older people often have problems with the practicalities of taking medicines and have compliance issues. In addition, people who are confused, depressed or have poor memories may have difficulty in taking medicines. The following principles may be helpful:

- A full medication history should be taken (including over-the-counter drugs) – this should highlight any previous adverse reactions, potential interactions, and any compliance issues.
- Keep the regime simple:
  - Use as few drugs as possible.
  - Note that compliance is better for drugs taken once or twice a day compared to three or four times a day.

- Be familiar with the drugs you prescribe.
- Ensure that the most suitable drug has been chosen for the patient.
- Ensure that the dose is correct. Start with a low dose and titrate slowly.
- Find out if the patient suffers from any other disease for which the drug is contraindicated.
- Consider the risk of drug interactions.
- Clear and simple instructions should be given to the patient, and the container must be clearly labelled. Many older people are unable to read leaflets and labels due to failing eyesight and may need specially written instructions.
- Various compliance aids are available, but it is important to establish that the patient can use them.
- Consider different formulations – liquids instead of large or small and fiddly tablets or capsules; combination products to reduce the number of medicines to take; slow-release preparations to reduce adverse effects.
- If an elderly patient develops sudden symptoms or changes in behaviour or condition, consider if this could be drug related.
- Review medication regularly – detailed medicines review can show that:
    - Some long-term treatments can be withdrawn – do not continue to use a drug for longer than necessary.
    - Some medicines are under-used.
    - Some medicines are not taken. As many as 50% of older people may not be taking their medicines as intended.

References

Anon. Office for National Statistics: www.statistics.gov.uk, accessed May 9, 2014.

Anon. Prescribing for the older person. *MeReC Bulletin* 2000; 11(10): 37–40.

Armour D, Cairns C. *Medicines in the Elderly* (2002). Pharmaceutical Press, London.

Department of Health (DH). The National Service Framework (NSF) – Medicines and Older People. London, March 2001.

Grahame-Smith DG, Aronson JK. *Oxford Textbook of Clinical Pharmacology and Drug Therapy* (2001). 3rd ed. Oxford University Press, Oxford.

Greenstein B, Gould D. *Trounce's Clinical Pharmacology for Nurses* (2004). 18th ed. Churchill Livingstone, Edinburgh.

Walker R, Whittlesea C (editors). *Clinical Pharmacy and Therapeutics* (2012). 5th ed. Churchill Livingstone, Oxford.

13 SOURCES AND INTERPRETATION OF DRUG INFORMATION

OBJECTIVES

At the end of this chapter, you should be familiar with the following:

- Sources of information
- The Internet
- Content of a summary of product characteristics (SPC)
- Content of a product information sheet

KEY POINTS

Sources of drug information

General

- *British National Formulary* (BNF)
- *British National Formulary for Children* (BNF-C)
- *Electronic Medicines Compendium* – information provided by drug companies about their products
- The Medicines and Healthcare Products Regulatory Agency (MHRA)

Specialist books

- *Neonatal Formulary: Drug Use in Pregnancy and the First Year of Life* – current edition
- *Paediatric Formulary* – Guy's, St. Thomas' and Lewisham Hospitals

Summary of product characteristics (SPC)

Information can be supplied by drug manufacturers in the form of a drug data sheet or summary of product characteristics (SPC). It provides essential information to ensure that the drug or medicine is used correctly, effectively and safely.

The information given in the SPC is also summarized in the package insert found inside the box. The package insert contains the basic information necessary for the administration and monitoring of the drug.

INTRODUCTION

Before administering any drug, you should have some idea of how that drug acts, its effect on the body, and possible side effects. This is certainly true when dealing with parenteral products as they will have a more immediate and dramatic effect compared to oral preparations.

Basic drug information can be found in reference books or, increasingly, from Web-based resources – many of the text-based resources are available online.

The following is a list of some sources of information. It is not meant to be exhaustive, but a list of resources that should be readily available on the ward, either as a book or via the Internet. The paediatric books should be available on paediatric wards, and if not, they will be available in the hospital pharmacy.

SOURCES OF DRUG INFORMATION

General

- *British National Formulary* (BNF) – current edition, Pharmaceutical Press, London
- *British National Formulary for Children* (BNF-C), Pharmaceutical Press, London
  Also available online at:
  http://www.medicinescomplete.com/mc/bnf/current/
  http://www.medicinescomplete.com/mc/bnfc/current/
  As a smart phone app via the National Institute for Health and Clinical Excellence (NICE) website:
  http://www.nice.org.uk/aboutnice/nicewebsitedevelopment/NICEApps.jsp
- Electronic Medicines Compendium – information provided by drug companies of their products: http://emc.medicines.org.uk/
- Drug package insert – if the drug is available in its original container, then there should be a package insert containing general information for that drug.
- The Medicines and Healthcare Products Regulatory Agency (MHRA) also provides information on all licensed drugs: http://www.mhra.gov.uk/spc-pil/

Specialist books

- *Neonatal Formulary: Drug Use in Pregnancy and the First Year of Life* – current edition, Northern Neonatal Network, Wiley-Blackwell. Updates are available from http://neonatalformulary.com
- *Paediatric Formulary* – current edition, Guy's, St. Thomas' and Lewisham Hospitals. Available from http://www.guysandstthomas.nhs.uk/resources/publications/formulary/paediatric-formulary-9th-edition.pdf

Your local hospital pharmacy department will be able to give advice on many aspects of dosing and administration of drugs.

THE INTERNET

The Internet is increasingly being used as a source for drug information, but care must be taken as to what information is used, as the validity and accuracy of some information may be suspect. The Internet should not be considered a first-line resource – established sources (such as reference books) should be used first. If the Internet is used, make sure the websites are reliable.

Internet warnings

When using the Internet, it is important to remember:

- The Internet is not owned by anybody or any organization.
- There are no restrictions on what is put onto the Internet and by whom.
- The Internet has no regard for geography – it can be just as easy to find information from the United Kingdom as it is to find information from abroad.
- The Internet is not a peer-reviewed source (although some individual websites might be).
- No UK body currently actively checks health information on the Internet.
- The Internet is an easy forum for distributing rumours and hoax information ('Internet Health Fraud').

Bearing in mind these warnings, as easily as you can find accurate information, you can find inaccurate information. Not all information sources are equally valuable or reliable. In comparison to traditional textbook information, there is a lack of publisher input associated with the Internet, and hence a lack of editorial review and adherence to standards.

In recognition of the problems of accuracy of information, NICE hosts the NHS Evidence website. NICE Evidence Services are a suite of services that provide Internet access to high-quality, authoritative evidence and best practice. The services cover health, social care and public health evidence. Evidence Services aim to help professionals make better and quicker evidence-based decisions.

In addition, anything with the following domain names are usually reliable sources of information:

- .nhs = National Health Service
- .ac = academic institution
- .gov = government department or agency

- .org = not-for-profit organization – examples include professional bodies (such as the RCN) and support or charity organizations (such as the British Heart Foundation)

Any information not from a recognized source should be assessed for quality before being used to influence patient care.

SUMMARY OF PRODUCT CHARACTERISTICS (SPC)

Before a drug is marketed, it is extensively researched and tested over many years. During this time, a great deal of information is gathered about efficacy, side effects and toxicology.

The most important information regarding the drug is documented in the Summary of Product Characteristics – the SPC, also called the data sheet – which is officially approved when the medicine is licensed for use. These can be viewed via the *Electronic Medicines Compendium* website (see list of sources of information on how to access SPCs and the MHRA websites).

The main purpose of an SPC is to provide essential information to ensure that the drug or medicine is used correctly, effectively and safely.

What an SPC contains

All SPCs are presented in the same way, using a standard heading for each section. The following list gives a brief description of these headings.

1. Name of the medicinal product
The trade or brand name of the drug or medicine.

2. Qualitative and quantitative composition
The generic or chemical names of the active ingredients and the amount of each active ingredient are provided, e.g. amount per tablet, amount per volume of solution, etc.

3. Pharmaceutical form
The form in which the medicine is presented, e.g. tablets, suppositories, ointment, etc.

4. Clinical particulars
How the medicine should be used – information is provided for pre-scribers to ensure that patients are treated appropriately, taking into account the patient's medical history, any other co-existing diseases or conditions, and other current treatments.

4.1 Therapeutic indications

The diseases or conditions that the medicine is licensed to treat are noted.

4.2 Posology and method of administration

Posology refers to the science of dosage, i.e. how much of a medicine should be given to a patient. The dose of the drug is given, including any changes in dose that may be necessary according to age or other disease or condition, such as renal or hepatic impairment. Where relevant, information is also given on the timing of doses in relation to meals.

The maximum single dose, the maximum daily dose and the maximum dose for a course of treatment may also be given.

4.3 Contraindications

Any information about a patient's condition, medical history or current treatments that may indicate that this medicine should not be given is provided.

4.4 Special warnings and special precautions for use

Any circumstances or conditions where the drug should be used with particular care are noted.

4.5 Interactions with other medicinal products and other forms of interaction

Any other medicines, or anything else that the patient is likely to take, which may react with the drug, for example, food or alcohol as well as other drugs, are provided.

4.6 Pregnancy and lactation

Advice is provided on the risks associated with using the drug at various stages of pregnancy and in fertile women, based upon the results of animal studies and any published observations in humans. If the drug or any of its metabolites are excreted in breast milk, the probability and nature of any adverse effects on the infant are described, and whether breast feeding should continue or not. The information is very limited – it is best to consult specialist textbooks or services (such as Medicine Information centres).

4.7 Effects on ability to drive and use machines

Whether or not the medicine is likely to impair a patient's ability to drive or operate machinery and if so, the extent of the effect is given.

4.8 Undesirable effects

A description of the side effects which may occur is provided, including how likely they are to happen, how severe they may be, and for how long they are likely to last. It should be borne in mind that the information presented is based on that gathered during clinical trials; patient numbers may be small and restricted, e.g. by age.

4.9 Overdose

A description is provided of the signs and symptoms of overdose, together with advice on how to treat.

5. Pharmacological properties

Information is provided about how the medicine works and how it is handled by the body.

5.1 Pharmacodynamic properties

How the medicine achieves, or is believed to achieve, its therapeutic effect in the body is presented.

5.2 Pharmacokinetic properties

Information is provided on how the medicine is taken up, distributed in the body and then removed. Where appropriate, additional information may be included as to how the pharmacokinetics may change according to, for example, the patient's age or state of health.

5.3 Preclinical safety data

This describes the effects of the drug that were observed in studies before being used in humans, which could be of relevance to the prescriber in assessing the risks and benefits of treatment.

6. Pharmaceutical particulars

Information is provided on the medicine ingredients, storage and packaging.

6.1 List of excipients

The contents of the medicine apart from the active ingredients, such as binding agents, solvents and flavourings are given.

6.2 Incompatibilities

In addition to the information given under *Interaction with Other Medicaments and Other Forms of Interaction*, information about any other medicines or materials that interact with the drug and with which it should therefore not be used or mixed.

6.3 Shelf life

This is the maximum length of time for which the medicine may be stored under the specified conditions and after which it should not be used.

6.4 Special precautions for storage

These are the conditions in which the medicine must be stored to avoid degradation, for example, excessive temperatures or light.

6.5 Nature and contents of container

A description is provided of the packaging and any other materials included in the pack, such as desiccants.

6.6 Special precautions for disposal and other handling

Instructions are provided for the preparation or administration of the medicine in addition to those given under *Posology and Method of Administration*. This section is particularly useful for information on the administration of parenteral drugs as it will give information on diluents, infusion fluids or stability.

7. Marketing authorization holder

This is the drug company holding the marketing authorization granted by the licensing authority.

8. Marketing authorization number

This is the licence number for the marketing authorization granted by the licensing authority.

9. Date of first authorization/renewal of authorization

This is the date when the marketing authorization was first granted. If the licence has at some time been suspended, the date when the licence was renewed is provided.

10. Date of (partial) revision of the text

This is the last date on which an alteration to the wording of the SPC was officially made to reflect, for example, the addition of a new therapeutic indication or a change to the pack sizes available.

The information given in the SPC is also summarized in the package insert found inside the box. The package insert contains the basic information necessary for the administration and monitoring of the drug.

As an example, let us look at the package insert for clarithromycin injection in more detail, as this is the usual form in which you are presented drug information. The important points to note would be as follows.

Administration information

Recommended administration

<u>Clarithromycin should not be given as a bolus or an intramuscular injection.</u>
Clarithromycin IV should be administered into one of the larger proximal veins as an IV infusion over 60 minutes, using a solution concentration of about 2 mg/mL.

STEP 1

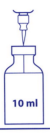

STEP 2

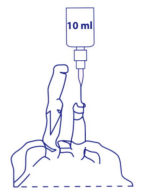

Add 10 mL sterilized Water for Injections into the vial and shake.
Use within 24 hours.
May be stored from 5°C up to room temperature.

Add 10 mL from Step 1 to 250 mL of a suitable diluent (see below).

This provides a 2 mg/mL solution.
Use within 6 hours (at room temperature) or within 24 hours if stored at 5°C.

DO NOT USE

- Diluents containing preservatives
- Diluents containing inorganic salts

DO NOT USE

- Solution strengths greater than 2 mg/mL (0.2%)
- Rapid infusion rates (<60 minutes)
- Failure to observe these precautions may result in pain along the vein

Administration

- Clarithromycin should not be given as an IV bolus or by IM injection – it must be given as an intermittent infusion.
- The infusion must be given over at least 60 minutes.
- The concentration of the infusion should not be greater than 2 mg/mL (0.2%); usually given in 250 mL.

Let us see how this is calculated:

Maximum concentration is 2 mg/mL, which is equal to:

$$1 \text{ mg in } \frac{1}{2} \text{ mL} = 0.5 \text{ mL}$$

Therefore, for a 500 mg dose = 500 × 0.5 = 250 mL.

So, the minimum volume for a 500 mg dose would be 250 mL.

Reconstitution information

- Water for Injection BP must be used.
- The volume for reconstitution is 10 mL.
- Once reconstituted, it must be used within 24 hours.
- Once added to the infusion bag, it must be used within 6 hours (24 hours if stored in a fridge).

Recommended diluents

Recommended diluents

5% dextrose in Lactated Ringer's solution, 5% dextrose, Lactated Ringer's solution, 5% dextrose in 0.3% sodium chloride, Normosol-M in 5% dextrose, Normosol-R in 5% dextrose, 5% dextrose in 0.45% sodium chloride, or 0.9% sodium chloride. Compatibility with other IV additives has not been established.

Suitable infusion fluids include sodium chloride 0.9% or 5% dextrose.

REVISION TEST

The purpose of this revision test is to re-assess your ability at drug calculations after you have finished the book.

You should get most, if not all, of the questions right. If you get wrong answers for any particular section, then you should go back and re-do that section, as this indicates that you have not fully understood that type of calculation.

SECTION ONE: BASICS

The aim of this section is see if you understand basic principles such as fractions, decimals, powers and using calculators.

Long multiplication

Solve the following:

1 567×405
2 265×2.45

Long division

Solve the following:

3 $4158 \div 21$
4 $26.88 \div 1.12$

Fractions

Solve the following, leaving your answer as a fraction:

5 $\dfrac{5}{16} \times \dfrac{4}{7}$

6 $\dfrac{4}{9} \times \dfrac{2}{3}$

7 $\dfrac{3}{8} \div \dfrac{6}{7}$

8 $\dfrac{2}{5} \div \dfrac{12}{15}$

Convert to a decimal (give answers to two decimal places):

9 $\dfrac{4}{7}$

10 $\dfrac{8}{18}$

Decimals

Solve the following:

11 2.15×0.64
12 $4.2 \div 0.125$
13 2.6×100
14 $45.67 \div 1{,}000$

Convert the following to a fraction:

15 0.4
16 0.025

Roman numerals

Write the following as ordinary numbers:

17 III
18 VII

Powers

Convert the following to a proper number:

19 2.3×10^2

Convert the following number to a power of 10:

20 800,000

PER CENT AND PERCENTAGES

This section is designed to see if you understand the concept of percent and percentages.

21 How much is 34% of 500 g?
22 What percentage is 220 g of 500 g?

UNITS AND EQUIVALENCES

This section is designed to re-test your knowledge on units, and how to convert from one unit to another.
    Convert the following.

Units of weight

23 0.125 milligrams (mg) to micrograms (mcg)
24 0.5 grams (g) to milligrams (mg)
25 250 nanograms (ng) to micrograms (mcg)

Units of volume

26 0.45 litres (L) to millilitres (mL)

Units of amount of substance

27 0.15 moles (mol) to millimoles (mmol)

DRUG STRENGTHS OR CONCENTRATIONS

This section is designed to see if you understand the various ways in which drug strengths can be expressed.

Percentage concentration

28 How much glucose (in grams) is there in a 500 mL infusion of glucose 10%?

mg/mL concentrations

29 What is the concentration (in mg/mL) of a 30% sodium chloride ampoule?

'I in …' concentrations or ratio strengths

30 You have a 1 mL ampoule of adrenaline/epinephrine 1 in 1,000. How much adrenaline/epinephrine (in milligrams) does the ampoule contain?

Parts per million (ppm) strengths

31 If a disinfectant solution contains 1,000 ppm of chlorine, how much chlorine (in milligrams) would be present in 5 litres?

DOSAGE CALCULATIONS

This is to test you on the type of calculations you will be doing every day on the ward. It includes dosage based on patient parameters and paediatric calculations.

Calculating the number of tablets or capsules required

The strength of the tablets or capsules you have available does not always correspond to the dose required. Therefore, you have to calculate the number of tablets or capsules needed.

32 Dose prescribed is lisinopril 15 mg. You have 5 mg tablets available. How many tablets do you need?

Drug dosage

Sometimes the dose is given on a body weight basis or in terms of body surface area. The following tests your ability at calculating doses on these parameters.

Work out the dose required for the following:

33 Dose = 7.5 mg/kg   Weight = 78 kg
34 Dose = 4 mcg/kg/min   Weight = 56 kg
35 Dose = 4.5 mg/m²   Surface area = 1.94 m²

(give answer to two decimal places)

Calculating dosages

Calculate how much you need for the following dosages

36 You have haloperidol injection 5 mg in 1 mL; amount required = 6 mg.
37 You have diazepam suspension 2 mg in 5 mL; amount required = 5 mg.
38 You have codeine phosphate syrup 25 mg in 5 mL; amount required = 30 mg.
39 You have co-trimoxazole injection 480 mg in 5 mL; amount required = 2,040 mg.

What volume and how many ampoules do you need?

Paediatric calculations

40 The dose of morphine for a 6-month-old child (7 kg) is 200 mcg/kg. How much do you need to draw up if morphine is available as a 10 mg/mL ampoule?

Other factors to take into account include displacement volumes for antibiotic injections.

41 A child is prescribed co-amoxiclav injection at a dose of 350 mg. The displacement volume for co-amoxiclav is 0.9 mL per 1.2 g vial. How much Water for Injections do you need to add to ensure a strength of 1.2 g per 20 mL?

Prescribing

42 You want to prescribe simple linctus 10 mL QDS for 2 weeks. Simple linctus is available as 200 mL bottles. How many bottles should be prescribed to ensure at least 2 weeks of treatment?
43 You want to prescribe co-codamol dispersible 8/500, 2 QDS for 5 days. Each 20-tablet pack costs £1.60. How much will it cost to prescribe treatment for 5 days?

INFUSION RATE CALCULATIONS

This section tests your knowledge of various infusion rate calculations. It is designed to see if you know the different drop factors for different giving sets and fluids, and if you are able to convert volumes to drops and vice versa.

Calculation of drip rates

44 What is the rate required to give 1 litre of sodium chloride 0.9% infusion over 8 hours using a standard giving set?

45 What is the rate required to give 1 unit of blood (500 mL) over 6 hours using a standard giving set?

Conversion of dosages to mL/hour

Sometimes it may be necessary to convert a dose (mg/min) to an infusion rate (mL/hour).

46 You have an infusion of dobutamine 250 mg in 250 mL. The dose required is 6 mcg/kg/min and the patient weighs 77 kg. What is the rate in mL/hour?

47 You are required to give a patient glyceryl trinitrate (50 mg in 50 mL) as a continuous infusion at a rate of 50 micrograms/min, at what rate should the infusion pump be set (mL/hour)?

Conversion of mL/hour back to a dose

48 You have enoximone 100 mg in 100 mL, and the rate at which the pump is running = 30 mL/hour. What dose is the pump delivering in mcg/kg/min?
(Patient's weight = 96 kg)

Calculating the length of time for IV infusions

49 A 1 litre infusion of sodium chloride 0.9% is being given at a rate of 28 drops/min (standard giving set).
How long will the infusion run at the specified rate?

50 A 500 mL infusion of glucose 5% is being given at a rate of 167 mL/hr.
How long will the infusion run at the specified rate?

COMPARE YOUR SCORES

	MARK OUT OF 50	%AGE SCORE (double the figure in the previous column)	DIFFERENCE (subtract the revision % from the pre-test % in the previous column)
Pre-test score			
Revision test score			

ANSWERS TO PROBLEMS

Basics

Long multiplication
1 229,635
2 649.25

Long division
3 198
4 24

Fractions
5 $\dfrac{5}{28}$

6 $\dfrac{8}{27}$

7 $\dfrac{7}{16}$

8 $\dfrac{1}{2}$

9 0.57

10 0.44

Decimals
11 1.376
12 33.6
13 260
14 0.04567
15 $\dfrac{2}{5}$

16 $\dfrac{1}{40}$

Roman numerals
17 3
18 7

Powers
19 230
20 8×10^5

Per cent and percentages

21 170 g
22 44%

Units and equivalences

Units of weight
23 125 micrograms
24 500 milligrams
25 0.25 micrograms

Units of volume
26 450 millilitres

Units of amount of substance
27 150 millimoles

Drug strengths or concentrations

Percentage concentration
28 50 g

mg/mL concentrations
29 300 mg/1 mL

'I in …' concentrations or ratio strengths
30 1 mg

Parts per million (ppm) strengths
31 5 mg

Dosage calculations

Calculating the number of tablets or capsules required
32 Three lisinopril 5 mg tablets

Drug dosage
33 585 mg
34 224 micrograms/min
35 8.730 mg

Calculating dosages
36 1.2 mL
37 12.5 mL
38 6 mL
39 21.25 mL and 5 ampoules

Paediatric calculations
40 0.14 mL
41 19.1 mL

Prescribing
42 Three 200 mL bottles (560 mL)
43 £3.20 (2 × 20 or £1.60)

Infusion rate calculations

Calculation of drip rates
44 41.7 drops/min (rounded to 42 drops/min)
45 20.8 drops/min (rounded to 21 drops/min)

Conversion of dosages to mL/hour
46 27.7(2) mL/hour
47 3 mL/hour

Conversion of mL/hour back to a dose
48 5.21 mcg/kg/min (approx. 5 mcg/kg/min)

Calculating the length of time for IV infusions
49 11.9 hours (approx. 12 hours)
50 2.99 hours (approx. 3 hours)

ANSWERS TO PROBLEMS

Here you will find the answers to the problems set in each chapter

Chapter 3 Per cent and percentages

Question 1   Before attempting the calculation, first estimate the answer.

The percentage is 30 which we can consider to be approximately one-third. To make the estimation easier, we will keep the number as 3,090 (as it is divisible by 3). So, we are now looking at one-third of 3,090 which is 1,030.

Alternatively, we can estimate the answer by manipulation of numbers.

Round down the amount to 3,000

100% – 3,000

10%   – 300 (by dividing by 10)

30%   – 900 (by multiplying by 3)

As the amount was rounded down, then the answer will be slightly higher – 920 would be a good guess.

Now we can attempt the calculation.

When doing percentage calculations, the number or quantity you want to find the percentage of is always equal to 100%.

So, 3.090 is equal to 100% and you want to find out how much 30% is.

Calculate how much is equal to 1%, i.e. divide by 100 (you are using the one unit rule)

$$1\% = \frac{3,090}{100}$$

Multiply by the percentage required (30%):

$$30\% = \frac{3,090}{100} \times 30 = 927$$

Checking the calculated answer of 927 with our estimation of 920 to 1,030 means that we should be confident in our calculated answer.

Answer: 30% of 3,090 = 927

We can use the formula:

$$part = \frac{whole}{100} \times percent$$

where:

whole = 3,090

percent = 30%

Substitute the numbers in the formula:

$$\frac{3,090}{100} \times 30 = 927$$

Answer: 30% of 3,090 = 927

Question 2   **Answer:** 35,973

Question 3   **Answer:** 450

Question 4   **Answer:** 48.36

Question 5   **Answer:** 150 mg

Question 6   Before attempting the calculation, first estimate the answer. Leave the numbers as they are both multiples of five and ten:

750 – 100%
150 – 20% (dividing by 5)
30   – 4% (dividing by 5)
60   – 8% (multiplying by 2)

Although we have calculated the answer needed, it is always a good idea to do the calculation to check that you have the right answer.

Now we can attempt the calculation.

The number or quantity you want to find the percentage of is always equal to 100%.

So, 750 would be equal to 100% and you want to find out the percentage of 60:

$$750 = 100\%$$

Calculate the percentage for 1, i.e. divide by 750 using the one unit rule:

$$1 = \frac{100\%}{750}$$

Multiply by the number you wish to find the percentage of, i.e. the smaller number (60):

$$60 = \frac{100}{750} \times 60 = 8\%$$

Checking the calculated answer of 8% with our estimation of 8% means that we should be confident in our calculated answer.

Answer: 60 is 8% of 750.

Using the formula:

$$\text{percent} = \frac{\text{part}}{\text{whole}} \times 100$$

where:
part = 60
whole = 750

Substitute the numbers in the formula:

$$\frac{60}{750} \times 100 = 8\%$$

Answer: 60 is 8% of 750.

Question 7   Answer: 84%

Question 8   Answer: 63%

Question 9   Answer: 28%

Question 10   Answer: Bags A = 65%
Bags B = 60%
Bags C = 64%
Bags D = 75%
Bags B should be replaced.

Chapter 4 Units and equivalences

For all problems, no estimations are really necessary except that it is a good idea to consider which units are to be converted. If you are converting from a **larger** unit to a **smaller** unit (i.e. 'heavier' to a 'lighter' unit) needing more, **multiply**. To do the reverse, **divide**.

Question 1   Answer: 12.5 grams

Question 2   Answer: 0.25 micrograms

Question 3   Answer: 3,200 millilitres

Question 4   Answer: 27.3 millimoles

Question 5   Answer: 3.75 kilograms

Question 6   Answer: 50,000 micrograms

Question 7   Answer: 0.025 kilograms

Question 8   Answer: 4,500 nanograms

The 10^{-6} is a power. The -6 indicates that it is a negative power, i.e. the number is divided by 10 six times.

In reality, we would move the decimal point six places to the left, i.e.:

$$4.5 = 0.0000045 \text{ g}$$

When converting from a larger unit to a smaller unit, you multiply by 1,000.

Thus for each conversion, multiply by 1,000, i.e. the decimal point moves three places to the right.

Then 0.0000045 g equals 0.0045 mg equals 4.5 micrograms equals 4,500 nanograms.

Question 9   Answer: 500 micrograms in 2 mL

To convert milligrams to micrograms, you are going from a larger unit to a smaller unit, so you multiply by 1,000:

$$0.25 \text{ mg} \times 1,000 = 250 \text{ micrograms}$$

Thus you have 250 micrograms in 1 mL.

Multiply by 2 to find out how much is in 2 mL, i.e.

$$250 \times 2 = 500 \text{ micrograms.}$$

Question 10   Answer: 100 micrograms in a 2 mL ampoule.

To convert milligrams to micrograms, you are going from a larger unit to a smaller unit, so multiply by 1,000:

$$0.05 \text{ mg} \times 1,000 = 50 \text{ micrograms}$$

Thus you have 50 micrograms in 1 mL, so to find out how much is in a 2 mL ampoule, multiply by 2:

$$50 \text{ micrograms} \times 2 = 100 \text{ micrograms}$$

Chapter 5 Moles and millimoles

Question 1   Sodium chloride 300 mg/mL, 10 mL

Molecular mass = 58.5

Before attempting the calculation, first estimate the answer.

As already stated: 1 millimole of sodium chloride yields 1 millimole of sodium.

So it follows that the amount (in milligrams) equal to 1 millimole of sodium chloride will give 1 milli-mole of sodium.

We have 300 mg/mL sodium chloride.

So, for 10 mL = 10 × 300 = 3,000 mg.

From tables: molecular mass of sodium chloride = 58.5; for ease of calculation, round up to 60 (i.e. 1 mmol = 60 mg).

It follows:

$$1 \text{ mg} = \frac{1}{60}$$

$$3,000 \text{ mg} = \frac{1}{60} \times 3,000 = \frac{300}{6} = 50 \text{ mmol}$$

As the amount for 1 mmol has been rounded up, then the actual answer should be slightly higher – 52 mmol is a good guess.

Now we can attempt the calculation.

One millimole of sodium chloride will give 1 millimole of sodium.

So the amount (in milligrams) for 1 millimole of sodium chloride will give 1 millimole of sodium.

From tables, the molecular mass of sodium chloride = 58.5.

So 58.5 mg of sodium chloride will give 1 millimole of sodium.

Thus it follows:

1 mg of sodium chloride will give $\frac{1}{58.5}$ millimoles of sodium

Now work out the total amount of sodium chloride in a 10 mL ampoule.

You have 300 mg/mL; thus for 10 mL:

$$300 \times 10 = 3,000 \text{ mg}$$

Next work out the number of millimoles for the infusion:

$$1 \text{ mg will give } \frac{1}{58.5} \text{ millimoles}$$

$$3,000 \text{ mg will give } \frac{1}{58.5} \times 3,000 = 51.28 \ (51) \text{ mmol}$$

Checking the calculated answer of 51 mmol with our estimate of 52 mmol means that we should be confident that our calculated answer is correct.

Answer: There are 51 mmol (approx) of sodium in a 10mL ampoule containing sodium chloride 300 mg/mL.

If using the formula:

$$\text{total number of millimoles} = \frac{\text{mg/mL}}{\text{mg of substance containing 1 mmol}} \times \text{volume (mL)}$$

where, in this case

 mg/mL = 300
 mg of substance containing 1 mmol = 58.5
 volume = 10

Substitute the numbers in the formula:

$$\frac{300}{58.5} \times 10 = 51.28 \,(51)\, \text{mmol}$$

Answer: There are 51 mmol (approx.) of sodium in a 10 mL ampoule containing sodium chloride 300 mg/mL.

Question 2 Sodium bicarbonate 8.4%, 200 mL

Molecular mass = 84

Before attempting the calculation, first estimate the answer.

As already stated: 1 millimole of sodium bicarbonate yields 1 millimole of sodium.

So it follows that the amount (in milligrams) equal to 1 millimole of sodium bicarbonate will give 1 millimole of sodium.

We have 8.4% sodium bicarbonate which is 8.4 g per 100 mL.

So, 200 mL = 8.4 × 2 = 16.8 g; for ease of calculation, round up to 17 g.

Convert grams to milligrams by multiplying by 1,000:

$$17 \times 1,000 = 17,000 \text{ mg.}$$

From tables: molecular mass of sodium chloride = 84; for ease of calculation, round up to 85 (i.e. 1 mmol = 85 mg).

It follows:

$$1 \text{ mg} = \frac{1}{85}$$

$$17,000 \text{ mg} = \frac{1}{85} \times 17,000 = \frac{17,000}{85} = 200 \text{ mmol}$$

As the strength of the infusion and the amount for 1 mmol has been increased, 200 mmol is a good guess.

Now we can attempt the calculation:

One millimole of sodium bicarbonate will give 1 millimole of sodium.

So the amount (in milligrams) for 1 millimole of sodium bicarbonate will give 1 millimole of sodium.

From tables, the molecular mass of sodium bicarbonate = 84.

So 84 mg of sodium bicarbonate will give 1 millimole of sodium.

Thus it follows:

1 mg of sodium bicarbonate will give $\dfrac{1}{84}$ millimoles of sodium

Now work out the total amount of sodium bicarbonate in a 200 mL infusion.

$$8.4\% = 8.4 \text{ g in } 100 \text{ mL}$$
$$= 8,400 \text{ mg in } 100 \text{ mL}$$

Thus for a 200 mL infusion, the amount equals:

$$\frac{8,400}{100} \times 200 = 16,800 \text{ mg}$$

Next work out the number of millimoles for the infusion:

$$1 \text{ mg will give } \frac{1}{84} \text{ millimoles}$$

$$16,800 \text{ mg will give } \frac{1}{84} \times 16,800 = 200 \text{ mmol}$$

Checking the calculated answer of 200 mmol with our estimate of 200 mmol means that we should be confident that our calculated answer is correct.

Answer: There are 200 mmol of sodium in a 200 mL infusion of sodium bicarbonate 8.4%.

A formula can be devised:

$$\frac{\text{total number}}{\text{of mmol}} = \frac{\text{percentage strength (\% w/v)}}{\text{mg of substance containing 1 mmol}} \times 10 \times \text{volume (mL)}$$

where in this case:

percentage strength (% w/v) = 8.4
mg of substance containing 1 mmol = 84
volume = 200

Substituting the numbers in the formula:

$$\frac{8.4}{84} \times 10 \times 200 = 200 \text{ mmol of sodium}$$

Answer: There are 200 mmol of sodium in a 200 mL infusion of sodium bicarbonate 8.4%.

Chapter 6 Drug strengths or concentrations

Question 1	0.9% w/v equals 0.9 g in 100 mL
	9 g in 1,000 mL (multiply by 10)
	Answer: 9 g
Question 2	Potassium 0.3% w/v equals 0.3 g in 100 mL
	3 g in 1,000 mL (multiply by 10)
	Sodium 0.18% w/v equals 0.18 g in 100 mL
	1.8 g in 1,000 mL (multiply by 10)
	Glucose 4% w/v equals 4 g in 100 mL
	40 g in 1,000 mL (multiply by 10)
	Answer: Potassium, 3 g; sodium, 1.8 g; glucose, 40 g
Question 3	0.45% w/v equals 0.45 g in 100 mL
	2.25 g in 500 mL (multiply by 5)
	Answer: 2.25 g
Question 4	Calcium gluconate 10% w/v is equal to: 10 g in 100 mL
	Therefore in a 10 mL ampoule, there is 1 g calcium gluconate.
	But you need 2 g, i.e. 2 ampoules = 2 g or 20 mL calcium gluconate 10%.
	Answer: You need to draw up 20 mL, which is equivalent to 2 ampoules.
Question 5	**Answer:** 4.5 mg/mL (multiply by 10)
Question 6	**Answer:** 5 mg/mL (multiply by 10)
Question 7	Potassium 2 mg/mL (multiply by 10)
	Sodium chloride 1.8 mg/mL (multiply by 10)
	Glucose 40 mg/mL (multiply by 10)
	Answer: Potassium, 2 mg/mL; sodium, 1.8 mg/mL; glucose, 40 mg/mL
Question 8	**Answer:** Bupivicaine 0.25% w/v (divide by 10)
Question 9	**Answer:** Glucose 50% w/v (divide by 10)
Question 10	Isosorbide dinitrate 0.05% w/v
	This last one is slightly different in that the strength given is in micrograms. So you have to convert this to milligrams by dividing by 1,000:

$$\frac{500}{1,000} = 0.5 \text{ mg}$$

Then divide by 10 as usual to give an answer of 0.05%.

Question 11 1 in 200,000 equals 1 g in 200,000 mL (or 1,000 mg in 20,000 mL)

Estimating the answer first:

We have: 200,000 mL – 1,000 mg

So: 200 mL – 1 mg   (dividing by 1,000)

It follows that: 20 mL – 0.1 mg   (dividing by 10)

Now calculate the answer to confirm your estimation.

1 in 200,000 equals 1 g in 200,000 mL (or 1,000 mg in 20,000 mL)

However, you have a 20 mL vial.

Next work out how many milligrams in 1 mL:

$$1\,mL = \frac{1,000}{200,000}\ mg\ \text{(using the one unit rule)}$$

Now work out how much is in the 20 mL vial:

$$20\,mL = \frac{1,000}{200,000} \times 20 = 0.1\,mg$$

Answer: There is 0.1 mg or 100 mcg of adrenaline/ epinephrine in a 20 mL vial containing 1 in 200,000.

Question 12 0.7 ppm means 0.7 g in 1,000,000 mL, or 0.7 mg in 1 litre

0.7 mg is equal to 700 micrograms

Answer: 700 micrograms per litre

Chapter 7 Dosage calculations

Calculating the number of tablets or capsules required

Question 1 Dose prescribed = 60 mg; tablets on hand are 15 mg and 30 mg

Before attempting the calculation, first estimate the answer.

First, check whether the dose prescribed and the medicine on hand are in the same units; in this case, both have the same units and so no conversion is needed.

Next, the dose prescribed (60 mg) is greater than the strength of both of the tablets on hand. We want to give as few a number of tablets as possible – so the higher strength of tablet is chosen.

Next, repeatedly add the strength for each tablet until you have reached the dose prescribed:

30 mg – one

60 mg – two

Although you have calculated the number of tablets needed, it is always a good idea to do the calculation to check that you have the right answer.

Now we can attempt the calculation:

Divide the dose needed (60 mg) by the strength of the tablet (30 mg).

Thus 60/30 = 2

Two tablets should be given.

Checking the calculated answer of 2 tablets with our estimate of 2 tablets means that we should be confident that our calculation is correct.

Answer: Two 30 mg tablets.

Question 2   Dose prescribed = 2.5 mg; tablets on hand are 0.5 mg, 1 mg, 3 mg and 5 mg

Before attempting the calculation, first estimate the answer.

First – check whether the dose prescribed and the medicine on hand are in the same units; in this case, both have the same units and so no conversion is needed.

Next – the dose prescribed (2.5 mg) is greater than the strength of the 0.5 mg and 1 mg tablets on hand, but less than the 3 mg and 5 mg tablets. We want to give as few a number of tablets as possible – so the lower strength of tablet is chosen.

Next, repeatedly add the strength for each tablet until you have reached the dose prescribed:

1 mg   –   one

2 mg   –   two

2.5 mg   –   two and a half

We could give a half a tablet, but we have a 0.5 mg tablet on hand, so it is better to give a whole tablet rather than a half. So we would give two 1 mg tablets and one 0.5 mg tablet.

Although you have calculated the number of tablets needed, it is always a good idea to do the calculation to check that you have the right answer.

Now we can attempt the calculation:

Divide the dose needed (2.5 mg) by the strength of the tablet (1 mg).

Thus $\dfrac{2.5}{1} = 2.5$

Two and a half 1 mg tablets should be given.

We could give a half a tablet, but we have a 0.5 mg tablet on hand, so it is better to give a whole tablet rather than a half. We would give two 1 mg tablets and one 0.5 mg tablet.

Checking the calculated answer of two 1 mg tablets and one 0.5 mg tablet with our estimate of two 1 mg tablets and one 0.5 mg tablet means that we should be confident that our calculation is correct.

Answer: Two 1 mg tablets and one 0.5 mg tablet

Question 3 Dose prescribed = 1 microgram; capsules on hand are 250 nanograms

Before attempting the calculation, first estimate the answer.

First, check whether the dose prescribed and the medicine on hand are in the same units; in this case, both have different units and so a conversion is needed.

Convert from micrograms to nanograms:

1 microgram = 1,000 nanograms

Each capsule contains 250 nanograms, so how many capsules contain 1,000 nanograms?

In this case, you can double the amount in each capsule until you have reached the dose prescribed:

    250 nanograms   – one
    500 nanograms   – two
    1,000 nanograms – four

Although you have calculated the number of capsules needed, it is always a good idea to do the calculation to check that you have the right answer.

Now we can attempt the calculation:

Divide the dose needed (1,000 nanograms) by the strength of the capsule (250 nanograms).

Thus $\dfrac{1,000}{250} = 4$

Four capsules should be given.

Checking the calculated answer of 4 capsules with our estimate of 4 capsules means that we should be confident that our calculation is correct.

Answer: Four 250 nanogram capsules

Dosages based on patient parameters

Question 4 Dose = 1.5 mg/kg. Patient's weight = 73 kg.

Before attempting the calculation, first estimate the answer.

First, round down the weight to 70 kg.

So 1.5 × 70 = 105 mg

As the weight used was rounded down, the actual dose will be slightly more – 110 mg would be a good guess.

Now we can attempt the calculation:

Therefore to calculate the total dose required, multiply:

$$1.5 \times 73 = 109.5$$

Thus you will need 109.5 mg (rounding up = 110 mg).

Checking the calculated answer of 110 mg with our estimate of 110 mg means that we should be confident that our calculation is correct.

Answer: 110 mg

Question 5 **Answer: 720 mg**

Question 6 **Answer: 97 mg**

Question 7 **Answer: 186 mg**

Question 8 **Answer: (a) 21,600 mcg; (b) 21.6 mg (22 mg)**

Question 9 **Answer: 325 mcg/min**

Question 10 Dose = 175 units/kg. Patient's weight = 74 kg.

The calculation is in two parts:

1. Calculation of dose required
2. Choice of syringe and the amount to administer based on the dose calculated

Calculation of dose required

Before attempting the calculation, first estimate the answer.

First, round up the weight to 75 kg.

To make calculations easier, split the weight into parts that are easy to calculate, i.e. in this case 50 kg and 25 kg.

For a dose of 175 units/kg = 175 × 50 = 8,750 units.

175 units/kg = 175 × 25 would be half of the above which equals 4,375 units.

Add the two together to give a total dose of 8,750 + 4,375 = 13,125 units.

As tinzaparin syringes are gradated in 1,000 units increments, it would be appropriate to round down to 13,000 units.

Now we can attempt the calculation:

Dose = 175 units/kg and the patient's weight = 74 kg

Therefore the dose required = 175 × 74 = 12,950 units

As tinzaparin syringes are gradated in 1,000 units increments, it would be appropriate to round up to 13,000 units.

Checking the calculated answer of 13,000 units with our estimate of 13,000 units means that we should be confident that our calculation is correct.

Choice of syringe and the amount to be administered

For a dose of 13,000 units, you will need a 0.7 mL (14,000 units) pre-filled syringe.

Before attempting the calculation, first estimate the answer.

We have: 14,000 units – 0.7 mL

So: 2,000 units – 0.1 mL   (dividing by 7)

So: 1,000 units – 0.05 mL   (dividing by 2)

Note – the above is equal to each graduation on each syringe.

It follows that 13,000 units – 0.65 mL (multiplying by 13).

Although we have calculated the dose needed, it is always a good idea to do the calculation to check that you have the right answer.

Now we can attempt the calculation:

Volume to be given: you have 14,000 units in 0.7 mL which is equivalent to

1 unit in $\dfrac{0.7}{14,000}$ mL

Therefore for 13,000 units, you will need:

$$\frac{0.7}{14,000} \times 13,000 = 0.65 \text{ mL}$$

Checking the calculated answer of 0.65 mL with our estimate of 0.65 mL means that we should be confident that our calculation is correct.

Answer: 13,000 units (0.65 mL) using a 14,000-units (0.7 mL) syringe

Question 11   Dose = 1.5 mg/kg. Patient's weight = 72 kg.

The calculation is in two parts:

1. Calculation of dose required
2. Choice of syringe and the amount to administer based on the dose calculated

Calculation of dose required

Before attempting the calculation, first estimate the answer.

First, round down the weight to 70 kg.

So $1.5 \times 70 = 105$ mg

Although the weight was rounded down, the estimated dose could be left as it is or be increased by 3 mg (graduations on the syringes).

Now we can attempt the calculation:

Therefore the dose required = $1.5 \times 72 = 108$ mg.

As enoxaparin syringes are gradated in 3 mg increments, it would be appropriate to maintain the dose at 108 mg as it is a multiple of 3.

Checking the calculated answer of 108 mg with our estimate of 105 mg means that we should be confident that our calculation is correct.

Choice of syringe and the amount to be administered

For a dose of 108 mg – you will need a 0.8 mL syringe (12,000 units, 120 mg).

Before attempting the calculation, first estimate the answer.

We have: 120 mg – 0.8 mL

So: 30 mg – 0.2 mL   (dividing by 4)

So: 3 mg – 0.02 mL   (dividing by 10)

Note – the above is equal to each gradation on each syringe.

It follows that 108 mg – 0.72 mL (multiplying by 36).

Although we have calculated the dose needed, it is always a good idea to do the calculation to check that you have the right answer.

Now we can attempt the calculation:

Volume to be given: you have 120 mg in 0.8 mL, which is equivalent to

$$1 \text{ mg in } \frac{0.8}{120} \text{ mL}$$

Therefore for 108 mg, you will need:

$$\frac{0.8}{120} \times 108 = 0.72 \text{ mL}$$

Checking the calculated answer of 0.72 mL with our estimate of 0.72 mL means that we should be confident that our calculation is correct.

Answer: 108 mg (0.72 mL) using a 120 mg (0.8 mL) syringe

Question 12   Using the formula:

$$m^2 = \sqrt{\frac{\text{height (cm)} \times \text{weight (kg)}}{3600}}$$

Height = 108 cm, weight = 20 kg, substitute the figures in the formula:

$$m^2 = \sqrt{\frac{108 \times 20}{3600}} \quad \text{Multiply the height by the weight}$$

$$m^2 = \sqrt{\frac{2160}{3600}} \quad \text{Divide the top line by the bottom line}$$

$$m^2 = \sqrt{0.6} = 0.77 \quad \text{Find the square root}$$
$$\text{Round the answer to two decimal places}$$

Answer: 0.77 m²

Question 13   Using the formula:

$$m^2 = \sqrt{\frac{\text{height (cm)} \times \text{weight (kg)}}{3600}}$$

Height = 180 cm, weight = 96 kg, substitute the figures in the formula:

$$m^2 = \sqrt{\frac{180 \times 96}{3600}} \quad \text{Multiply the height by the weight}$$

$$m^2 = \sqrt{\frac{17280}{3600}} \quad \text{Divide the top line by the bottom line}$$

$$m^2 = \sqrt{4.8} = 2.19 \quad \text{Find the square root}$$
$$\text{Round the answer to two decimal places}$$

Answer: 2.19 m²

Calculating drug dosages

Question 14 You have: erythromycin suspension 250 mg/5 mL
The dose required is 1 g.

Before attempting the calculation, first estimate the answer.

First, check whether the dose prescribed and the medicine on hand are in the same units; in this case, both have different units and so a conversion is needed.

We need to convert to the same units – convert the dose to milligrams as the units of the medicine on hand are in milligrams. Dose prescribed is 1 g which is equal to 1,000 mg.

The dose required of 1 g (1,000 mg) is more than the strength of the medicine on hand – so the answer will be more than 5 mL.

We have: 250 mg – 5 mL
So: 500 mg – 10 mL (by doubling)
It follows that: 1,000 mg – 20 mL (by doubling)

Although you have calculated the amount needed, it is always a good idea to do the calculation to check that you have the right answer.

Now we can attempt the calculation:

$$1 \text{ mg of suspension} = \frac{5}{250} \text{ mL (using the one unit rule)}$$

$$\text{Dose} = 1,000 \text{ mg} \left(1 \text{ g}\right), \text{ which will equal: } 1,000 \times \frac{5}{250} = 20 \text{ mL}$$

Checking the calculated answer of 20 mL with our estimate of 20 mL means that we should be confident that our calculation is correct.

Answer: 20 mL of erythromycin suspension 250 mg/5 mL is required

Question 15 You have: digoxin liquid 50 micrograms/mL
The dose required is 62.5 micrograms.

Before attempting the calculation, first estimate the answer.

Both the prescribed dose and the medicine on hand are in the same units – so there is no conversion needed.

The dose required of 62.5 micrograms is more than the strength of the medicine on hand – so the answer will be more than 1 mL.

We have: 50 micrograms – 1 mL
So: 10 micrograms – 0.2 mL (dividing by 5)
It follows: 60 micrograms – 1.2 mL (multiplying by 6)
The actual dose of 62.5 micrograms is slightly more – so a volume of 1.3 mL would be a good guess.

Now we can attempt the calculation:

$$1 \text{ microgram of liquid} = \frac{1}{50} \text{ mL} \quad \left(\text{using the one unit rule}\right)$$

$$\text{dose} = 62.5 \text{ micrograms, which will equal: } 62.5 \times \frac{1}{50} = 1.25 \text{ mL}$$

Checking the calculated answer of 1.25 mL with our estimate of 1.3 mL means that we should be confident that our calculation is correct.

Answer: 1.25 mL of digoxin liquid 50 micrograms/mL is required.

Question 16 You have: Oramorph® liquid 100 mg/5 mL.

The dose required is 60 mg.

Before attempting the calculation, first estimate the answer.

Both the prescribed dose and the medicine on hand are in the same units – so there is no conversion needed.

The dose required of 60 mg is less than the strength of the medicine on hand – so the answer will be less than 5 mL.

We have: 100 mg – 5 mL
So: 10 mg – 0.5 mL   (dividing by 10)
It follows: 60 mg – 3 mL   (multiplying by 6)

Although you have calculated the amount needed, it is always a good idea to do the calculation to check that you have the right answer.

Now we can attempt the calculation:

$$1 \text{ mg of liquid} = \frac{5}{100} \text{ mL} \left(\text{using the one unit rule}\right)$$

$$\text{dose} = 60 \text{ mg, which will equal: } 60 \times \frac{5}{100} = 3 \text{ mL}$$

Checking the calculated answer of 3 mL with our estimate of 3 mL means that we should be confident that our calculation is correct.

Answer: 3 mL of Oramorph liquid 100 mg/5 mL is required.

Question 17   You have: pethidine injection 100 mg/2 mL

Dose required = 75 mg

Before attempting the calculation, first estimate the answer.

Both the prescribed dose and the medicine on hand are in the same units – so there is no conversion needed.

The dose required of 75 mg is less than the strength of the medicine on hand – so the answer will be less than 2 mL.

We have: 100 mg – 2 mL
So: 50 mg – 1 mL   (by halving)
So: 25 mg – 0.5 mL   (by halving)

It follows: 75 mg – 1.5 mL   (by adding the above together – 50 mg + 25 mg or 1 mL + 0.5 mL)

Although you have calculated the amount needed, it is always a good idea to do the calculation to check that you have the right answer.

Now we can attempt the calculation:

$$\text{1 mg of injection} = \frac{2}{100}\text{ mL} \quad \left(\text{using the one unit rule}\right)$$

$$\text{dose} = 75\text{ mg, which will equal: } 75 \times \frac{2}{100} = 1.5\text{ mL}$$

Checking the calculated answer of 1.5 mL with our estimate of 1.5 mL means that we should be confident that our calculation is correct.

Answer: 1.5 mL of pethidine injection 100 mg/2 mL is required.

Question 18   Dose = 2 mg/kg   Weight = 23 kg

There is no need to estimate the dose required as it is a simple sum.

Dose required = dose × weight = 2 × 23 = 46 mg
You have ranitidine liquid = 150 mg in 10 mL
Dose required = 46 mg

Before attempting the calculation, first estimate the answer.

Both the prescribed dose and the medicine on hand are in the same units – so there is no conversion needed.

The dose required of 46 mg is less the strength of the medicine on hand – so the answer will be less than 10 mL.

For ease of calculation, round up the dose to 50 mg.
We have 150 mg – 10 mL

It follows that 50 mg – 3.3 mL (dividing by 3)

The actual dose of 46 mg is slightly less – so a volume of 3 mL would be a good guess.

Now we can attempt the calculation:

Therefore for 46 mg you will need: $\dfrac{10}{150} \times 46 =$

3.07 mL = 3 mL (rounded down).

Sometimes it is necessary to 'adjust' the dose like this for ease of calculation and administration, as long as the 'adjustment' is not so much as to make a large difference in the dose.

Checking the calculated answer of 3 mL with our estimate of 3 mL means that we should be confident that our calculation is correct.

Answer: You need to give 3 mL of ranitidine liquid 150 mg in 10 mL.

Question 19   Dose = 4 mg/kg   Weight = 18.45 kg

The calculation is in two parts:
1. Calculation of dose required
2. Volume of medicine to give based on the dose calculated

Calculation of dose required
Before attempting the calculation, first estimate the answer.

Round up the weight to 20 kg

So dose required would equal $4 \times 20 = 80$ mg

As the weight used was rounded up, the actual dose will be slightly less – 75 mg would be a good guess.

Total amount required = wgt × dose = 18.45 × 4 = 73.8 mg

Checking the calculated answer of 73.8 mg with our estimate of 75 mg means that we should be confident that our calculation is correct.

Volume of medicine to be administered
Before attempting the calculation, first estimate the answer.

You have: trimethoprim suspension 50 mg/5 mL

Dose required = 73.8 mg

Both the prescribed dose and the medicine on hand are in the same units – so there is no conversion needed.

The dose required of 73.8 mg is more than the strength of the medicine on hand – so the answer will be more than 5 mL.

We have 50 mg – 5 mL

So 25 mg – 2.5 mL (by halving)

It follows that 75 mg – 7.5 mL (by adding the above together – 50 mg + 25 mg or 5 mL + 2.5 mL).

The actual dose of 73.8 mg is slightly less – so a volume of 7.4 mL would be a good guess.

Now we can attempt the calculation:

$$1 \text{ mg of suspension} = \frac{5}{50} \text{ mL (using the one unit rule)}$$

$$\text{dose} = 73.8 \text{ mg, which will equal: } 73.8 \times \frac{5}{50} = 7.4 \text{ mL}$$

Checking the calculated answer of 7.4 mL with our estimate of 7.4 mL means that we should be confident that our calculation is correct.

Answer: 7.4 mL of trimethoprim suspension 50 mg/5 mL is required

Question 20   The prescribed dose is 2.5 mg/kg daily in two divided doses.

Weight = 68 kg

Before attempting the calculation, first estimate the answer.

Round up the weight to 70 kg

So 2.5 × 70 = 175 mg

As the weight used was rounded up, the actual dose will be slightly less – 170 mg would be a good guess.

This has to be given in two divided doses, so for each dose = $\frac{170}{2}$ = 85 mg.

Now we can attempt the calculation:

The patient weighs 68 kg, so the total daily dose (TDD) = 2.5 × 68 = 170 mg.

Checking the calculated answer of 170 mg with our estimate of 170 mg means that we should be confident that our calculation is correct.

This has to be given in two divided doses, so for each dose $= \dfrac{170}{2} = 85$ mg.

The capsules are available in 10 mg, 25 mg, 50 mg and 100 mg strengths, so you will need to give:

1 × 50 mg

1 × 25 mg

1 × <u>10 mg</u> +

85 mg

Question 21   Answer: Dose required = 76 × 5 = 380 mg, you will need two vials of 250 mg.

Question 22   Dose required for the patient = 50 × 0.5 = 25 mg/hour

There is no need to estimate the dose required as it is a simple sum.

Therefore for 12 hours, you will need: 25 × 12 = 300 mg

You have 250 mg in 10 mL

Dose required = 300 mg

Both the prescribed dose and the medicine on hand are in the same units – so there is no conversion needed.

Before attempting the calculation, first estimate the answer.

The dose required of 300 mg is more than the strength of the medicine on hand – so the answer will be more than 10 mL.

We have: 250 mg – 10 mL

So: 50 mg – 2 mL   (dividing by 5)

It follows: 300 mg – 12 mL   (multiplying by 6)

Although you have calculated the amount needed, it is always a good idea to do the calculation to check that you have the right answer.

Now we can attempt the calculation:

You have: 250 mg in 10 mL

Therefore: 1 mg would equal $\dfrac{10}{250}$ mL (using the one unit rule)

Thus: 300 mg $= \dfrac{10}{250} \times 300 = 12$ mL

Checking the calculated answer of 12 mL with our estimate of 12 mL means that we should be confident that our calculation is correct.

Answer: 12 mL

Question 23   This calculation is in four parts:

1. Volume of co-trimoxazole needed for each dose
2. Number of ampoules needed for each dose
3. Number of ampoules needed for 3 days
4. Choice of infusion bag

Volume needed for each dose

Total daily dose = 120 mg/kg and weight = 78 kg

Total daily dose is to be given in 4 divided doses; so each dose is equal to 120 mg

You have co-trimoxazole 96 mg/mL, 5 mL ampoules

Each ampoule contains 96 × 5 = 480 mg (480 mg/5 mL)

Before attempting the calculation, first estimate the answer.

Round up the weight to 80 kg and the strength of co-trimoxazole to 100 mg/mL.

So 120 × 80 = 9,600 mg

As the weight used was rounded up, the actual dose will be slightly less (2 lots of 120) – 9,400 mg would be a good guess.

We have: 100 mg – 1 mL

So: 400 mg – 4 mL   (multiplying by 4)

So: 900 mg – 9 mL   (multiplying by 9)

So: 9,000 mg – 90 mL (multiplying by 10)

It follows: 9,400 mg – 94 mL (by adding the above together – 9,000 mg + 400 mg or 90 mL + 4 mL)

Now we can attempt the calculation:

$$\text{total daily dose} = \text{wgt} \times \text{dose} = 120 \times 78 = 9{,}360 \text{ mg}$$

Checking the calculated answer of 9,360 mg with our estimate of 9,400 mg means that we should be confident that our calculation is correct.

Next we need to calculate the volume of co-trimoxazole 96 mg/mL (480 mg/5 mL) to draw up for our calculated dose.

Thus $1 \text{ mg} = \dfrac{1}{96} \text{ mL}$

Therefore for 9,360 mg you will need:

$$\frac{1}{96} \times 9{,}360 = 97.5 \text{ mL}$$

Checking the calculated answer of 97.5 mL with our estimate of 94 mL means that we should be confident that our calculation is correct.
Answer: 97.5 mL

Number of ampoules needed for each dose
The total daily dose (9,360 mg) is to be given in 4 divided doses.

Before attempting the calculation, first estimate the answer.

Both the prescribed dose and the medicine on hand are in the same units – so there is no conversion needed.

Round up the dose to 10,000 mg and the co-trimoxazole ampoule to 500 mg

As the total daily dose is to be given in four divided doses – divide by 4

Each dose = $\dfrac{10,000}{4}$ = 2,500 mg

Number of ampoules needed = $\dfrac{2,500}{500}$ = 5

Now we can attempt the calculation:
Therefore for each dose, you will need:

$$\frac{9,360}{4} = 2,340 \text{ mg}$$

You have co-trimoxazole ampoules containing 480 mg (480 mg/5 mL)

Number of ampoules needed = $\dfrac{2,340}{4}$ = 4.875

Obviously, we need 4 and a bit ampoules – so round up to five ampoules

Checking the calculated answer of 5 ampoules with our estimate of 5 ampoules means that we should be confident that our calculation is correct.
Answer: 5 ampoules

Number of ampoules needed for 3 days
We need 5 ampoules for each dose, so it follows:
5 ampoules – per dose
20 ampoules – per day (multiply by 4)
60 ampoules – for 3 days (multiply by 3)
Answer: 60 ampoules

Infusion of each dose
1 ampoule must be diluted to 125 mL

For the dose of 2,340 mg just over 4 ampoules were needed (4.875 ampoules) – so round up to five ampoules.

Five ampoules are needed for each dose: 5 × 125 mL = 625 mL

The nearest size of infusion bag available would be 1 litre

Answer: 1 litre sodium chloride 0.9%

Displacement volumes or values

Question 24

(i) Displacement volume = 0.8 mL per 1 g vial

Work out how much Water for Injections you need to add to make a final volume of 10 mL, i.e.

$$10 \text{ mL} - 0.8 \text{ mL} = 9.2 \text{ mL}$$

Therefore you need to add 9.2 mL Water for Injection to each vial to give a final concentration of 1 g/10 mL.

Now you have a final concentration of 100 mg/mL (1 g or 1,000 mg/10 mL).

(ii) The next step is to calculate the volume for 350 mg.

Before attempting the calculation, first estimate the answer.

We have 100 mg in 1 mL

Both the prescribed dose and the medicine on hand are in the same units – so there is no conversion needed.

The dose required of 350 mg is more than the strength of the medicine on hand – so the answer will be more than 1 mL

We have: 100 mg – 1 mL

So: 50 mg – 0.5 mL   (by halving)

So: 300 mg – 3 mL   (multiplying by 3)

It follows: 350 mg – 3.5 mL   (by adding the above together – 300 mg + 50 mg or 3 mL + 0.5 mL)

Although you have calculated the amount needed, it is always a good idea to do the calculation to check that you have the right answer.

Now we can attempt the calculation:

We have 100 mg in 1 mL

So 1 mg = $\dfrac{1}{100}$ (using the one unit rule)

$$350 \text{ mg} = \frac{1}{100} \times 350 = 3.5 \text{ mL}$$

Checking the calculated answer of 3.5 mL with our estimate of 3.5 mL means that we should be confident that our calculation is correct.

Answer: You need to draw up a dose of 3.5 mL (350 mg).

(i) Displacement value = 0.5 mL for 1 g

Work out how much Water for Injections you need to add to make a final volume of 4 mL, i.e.

$$4 \text{ mL} - 0.5 \text{ mL} = 3.5 \text{ mL}$$

Therefore you need to add 3.5 mL Water for Injection to each vial to give a final concentration of 250 mg/mL.

Now you have a final concentration of 250 mg/mL (1 g or 1,000 mg/4 mL).

(ii) The next step is to calculate the dose:

Dose = 150 mg/kg. Patient's weight = 18 kg.

Before attempting the calculation, first estimate the answer.

Round up the weight to 20 kg

So 150 × 20 = 3,000 mg

As the weight used was rounded up, the actual dose will be slightly less – 2,800 mg would be a good guess.

As the total dose is to be given in four divided doses – divide by 4.

Each dose = $\dfrac{2,800}{4}$ = 700 mg

We have 1,000 mg in 4 mL

Both the prescribed dose and the medicine on hand are in the same units – so there is no conversion needed.

The dose required of 700 mg is less than the strength of the medicine on hand – so the answer will be less than 4 mL.

We have: 1,000 mg – 4 mL

So: 100 mg – 0.4 mL   (dividing by 10)

It follows: 700 mg – 2.8 mL   (multiplying by 7)

Now we can attempt the calculation:

total daily dose = wgt × dose = 18 × 150 = 2,700 mg

Checking the calculated answer of 2,700 mg with our estimate of 2,800 mg means that we should be confident that our calculation is correct.

As the total dose is to be given in four divided doses – divide by 4.

Each dose $= \dfrac{2,700}{4} = 675$ mg

We have 250 mg in 1 mL

So 1 mg $= \dfrac{1}{250}$ (using the one unit rule)

$$675 \text{ mg} = \frac{1}{50} \times 675 = 2.7 \text{ mL}$$

Checking the calculated answer of 2.7 mL with our estimate of 2.8 mL means that we should be confident that our calculation is correct.

Answer: You need to draw up a dose of 2.7 mL (675 mg).

Question 26

(i) Displacement value = 0.2 mL for 250 mg

Work out how much Water for Injections you need to add to make a final volume of 5 mL, i.e.

$$5 \text{ mL} - 0.2 \text{ mL} = 4.8 \text{ mL}$$

Therefore you need to add 4.8 mL Water for Injection to each vial to give a final concentration of 50 mg/mL.

Now you have a final concentration of 50 mg/mL (250 mg/5 mL).

(ii) The next step is to calculate the dose:

Dose = 12.5 mg/kg. Patient's weight = 19.6 kg.

Before attempting the calculation, first estimate the answer.

Round up the dose to 13 mg/kg and the weight to 20 kg

So 13 × 20 = 260 mg

As both the dose and weight used were rounded up, the actual dose will be slightly less – 250 mg would be a good guess.

We have 250 mg in 5 mL

Both the prescribed dose and the medicine on hand are in the same units – so there is no conversion needed.

The dose required of 250 mg is the same as the strength of the medicine on hand – so the answer will be 5 mL.

Now we can attempt the calculation:

total daily dose = wgt × dose = 19.6 × 12.5 = 245 mg

Checking the calculated answer of 245 mg with our estimate of 250 mg means that we should be confident that our calculation is correct.

We have 50 mg in 1 mL

Both the prescribed dose and the medicine on hand are in the same units – so there is no conversion needed.

So 1 mg = $\dfrac{1}{50}$ mL (using the one unit rule).

$$245 \text{ mg} = \dfrac{1}{50} \times 245 = 4.9 \text{ mL}$$

Checking the calculated answer of 4.9 mL with our estimate of 5 mL means that we should be confident that our calculation is correct.

Answer: You need to draw up a dose of 4.9 mL (245 mg).

Prescriber calculations

Question 27 This is a straightforward calculation, so estimation is not really needed.

Dose required = 30 mg QDS for 2 weeks; you have: codeine syrup 25 mg/5 mL

First, convert the amount required to a volume (to enable you to determine the volume needed for the total course).

1 mg of liquid = $\dfrac{5}{25}$ mL (using the one unit rule)

Dose = 30 mg, which will equal: $30 \times \dfrac{5}{25} = 6$ mL

Next, calculate how much is needed per day.

Dose = 6 mL (30 mg) QDS or 6 mL four times a day; dose per day equals

$$6 \times 4 = 24 \text{ mL}$$

Next, calculate the amount for the treatment course (2 weeks or 14 days):

$$24 \times 14 = 363 \text{ mL}$$

Each bottle is available as a 100 mL bottle, so the number needed equals

$$\frac{336}{100} = 3.36 \text{ bottles}$$

Round up to the nearest 'bottle' to ensure a sufficient amount for the desired treatment course.

Answer: Prescribe four 100 mL bottles.

Question 28   You want to prescribe a reducing dose of prednisolone. Starting at 20 mg daily for a week, then reducing by 5 mg every week to a dose of 5 mg daily for a week, then reducing by 1 mg every 2 days until zero milligrams is reached.

How many 5 mg and 1 mg tablets do you need to prescribe?

Once again, this is a straightforward calculation; you are simply counting the number of tablets needed.

To make this easier, write the dosing schedule needed:

20 mg daily for 1 week
15 mg daily for 1 week
10 mg daily for 1 week
5 mg daily for 1 week
4 mg daily for 2 days
3 mg daily for 2 days
2 mg daily for 2 days
1 mg daily for 2 days
STOP

Now that we know the regimen needed, we can now calculate the number of tablets needed for each strength:

20 mg daily for 1 week	Four 5 mg tablets per day; $4 \times 7 = 28$	Running total = 28 tablets
15 mg daily for 1 week	Three 5 mg tablets per day; $3 \times 7 = 21$	Running total = 49 tablets
10 mg daily for 1 week	Two 5 mg tablets per day; $2 \times 7 = 14$	Running total = 63 tablets
5 mg daily for 1 week	One 5 mg tablet per day; $1 \times 7 = 7$	Running total = 70 tablets

Continued

4 mg daily for 2 days	Four 1 mg tablets per day; $4 \times 2 = 8$	Running total = 8 tablets
3 mg daily for 2 days	Three 1 mg tablets per day; $3 \times 2 = 6$	Running total = 14 tablets
2 mg daily for 2 days	Two 1 mg tablets per day; $2 \times 2 = 4$	Running total = 18 tablets
1 mg daily for 2 days	One 1 mg tablet per day; $1 \times 2 = 2$	Running total = 20 tablets

Answer: You need to prescribe 70 × 5 mg tablets and 20 × 1 mg tablets.

Question 29   You want to prescribe an antacid to a patient at a dose of 10 mL at QDS for 28 days. Two brands are available:

Brand A costs £4.20 per 300 mL bottle and
Brand B costs £5.20 per 500 mL bottle.

This is a straightforward calculation, so estimation is not really needed.

First, calculate how much is needed per day:
Dose = 10 mL QDS or 10 mL four times a day; dose per day equals:

$$10 \times 4 = 40 \text{ mL}$$

Next, calculate the amount for the treatment course (28 days):

$$40 \times 28 = 1{,}120 \text{ mL}$$

For Brand A
Each bottle is available as a 300 mL bottle, so the number needed equals:

$$\frac{1{,}120}{300} = 3.73 \text{ bottles}$$

Round up to the nearest 'bottle' to ensure a sufficient amount for the desired treatment course.

Four 300 mL bottles are needed.

Cost of each bottle = £4.20, so four bottles will cost:

$$4 \times £4.20 = £16.80$$

For Brand B
Each bottle is available as a 500 mL bottle, so the number needed equals:

$$\frac{1,120}{500} = 2.24 \text{ bottles}$$

Round up to the nearest 'bottle' to ensure a sufficient amount for the desired treatment course.

Three 500 mL bottles are needed.

Cost of each bottle = £5.20, so three bottles will cost:

$$3 \times £5.20 = £15.60$$

So, it is more cost-effective to prescribe *Brand B*
Answer: Prescribe three 500 mL *Brand B* bottles.

Question 30 The current *British National Formulary* (BNF – No. 68) states:

Neuropathic pain, adult over 18 years, 300 mg once daily on day 1, then 300 mg twice daily on day 2, then 300 mg 3 times daily on day 3 *or* initially 300 mg 3 times daily on day 1, then increased according to response in steps of 300 mg (in 3 divided doses) every 2 to 3 days up to a maximum 3.6 g daily.

The first regimen appears to be the most appropriate:

Day 1 = one 300 mg capsule (300 mg once daily)
Day 2 = two 300 mg capsules (300 mg twice daily)
Running total = 3
Day 3 = three 300 mg capsules (300 mg three times daily)
Running total = 6
Day 4 to 14 (11 days) = thirty-three 300 mg capsules (300 mg three times daily)
Running total = 39

After 2 weeks, you decide to review the patient and re-assess the dose and increase if necessary.

Answer: Prescribe 33 × 300 mg gabapentin capsules.

Chapter 8 Infusion rate calculations

Calculating IV infusion rates (drops/min)

Question 1   Before attempting the calculation, first estimate the required drip rate.

You have 500 mL to be given over 6 hours – convert hours to minutes = 6 × 60 = 360 min (round up the time to 400 min).

Convert the infusion to a number of drops:

$$500 \times 20 = 10,000 \text{ drops}$$

So 10,000 drops to be given over 400 mins.

Therefore drops per minute would equal $\dfrac{10,000}{400} = \dfrac{100}{4} = 25$ drops/min.

As the length of time for the infusion was rounded up, then the actual drip rate will be slightly higher – around 27 drops/min would be a good guess.

Now we can attempt the calculation:

First convert the volume to a number of drops. To do this, multiply the volume of the infusion by the number of drops per mL for the giving set, i.e. 500 × 20 = 10,000 drops.

Next convert hours to minutes by multiplying the number of hours the infusion is to be given by 60 (60 minutes = 1 hour):

$$6 \text{ hours} = 6 \times 60 = 360 \text{ minutes}$$

Write down what you have just calculated, i.e. the total number of drops to be given over how many minutes:

$$10,000 \text{ drops} = 360 \text{ minutes}$$

Calculate the number of drops per minute by dividing the number of drops by the number of minutes, i.e. divide 10,000 by 360.

You have 10,000 drops over 360 minutes.

Thus drops/min $= \dfrac{10,000}{360} = 27.78$ drops/min

(28 drops/min, approx.)

Checking the calculated answer of 28 drops/min with our estimate of 27 drops/min would be a good guess. This means that we should be confident that our calculated answer is correct.

Answer: To give 500 mL of sodium chloride 0.9% over 6 hours, the rate will have to be 28 drops/min using a standard giving set (20 drops/mL).

If using the formula:

$$\text{drops/min} = \frac{\text{drops/mL of the giving set} \times \text{volume of the infusion}}{\text{number of hours the infusion is to run} \times 60}$$

where in this case:

drops/mL of the giving set = 20 drops/mL (SGS)
volume of the infusion (in mL) = 500 mL
number of hours the infusion is to run = 6 hours

Substitute the numbers in the formula:

$$\text{drops/min} = \frac{20 \times 500}{6 \times 60} = 27.78 \text{ drops/min (28 drops/min, approx.)}$$

Answer: To give 500 mL of sodium chloride 0.9% over 6 hours, the rate will have to be 28 drops/min using a standard giving set (20 drops/mL).

Question 2   27.7 drops/min (28 drops/min) – SGS (20 drops/mL)
Question 3   20.8 drops/min (21 drops/min) – SGS (15 drops/mL)

Conversion of dosages to mL/hour

Question 4   Glyceryl trinitrate 50 mg in 500 mL
Dose = 10 mcg/min

Before attempting the calculation, first estimate the required infusion rate.

Dose required = 10 mcg/min – find the amount per hour (by multiplying by 60) = 10 × 60 = 600 mcg/hour.

As the dose and drug are in different units, convert to the same units (convert milligrams to micrograms):

$$50 \text{ mg} = 50 \times 1{,}000 = 50{,}000 \text{ mcg}$$

We have an infusion containing:

50,000 mcg – 500 mL
1,000 mcg – 10 mL (dividing by 50)
100 mcg – 1 mL (dividing by 10)
600 mcg – 6 mL (multiplying by 6)

Infusion rate would be 6 mL/hour.

Although you have calculated the infusion rate required, it is always a good idea to do the calculation to check that you have the right answer.

Now we can attempt the calculation:

Dose = 10 mcg/min. The final answer is in terms of hours, so multiply by 60 to convert minutes into hours:

dose = 10 mcg/min = 10 × 60 = 600 mcg/hour

Convert mcg to mg by dividing by 1,000:

$$\frac{600}{1,000} = 0.6 \text{ mg/hour}$$

The next step is to calculate the volume for the dose required.

Calculate the volume for 1 mg of drug.

You have: 50 mg in 500 mL

$$1\,mg = \frac{500}{50} = 10\,mL$$

Thus for the dose of 0.6 mg, the volume is equal to: 0.6 mg = 0.6 × 10 = 6 mL/hour.

Checking the calculated answer of 6 mL/hour with our estimate of 6 mL/hour means that we should be confident that our calculated answer is correct.

Answer: The rate required = 6 mL/hour

As the dose is being given as a total dose (not on a weight basis), the following formula is used:

$$mL/hour = \frac{\text{volume to be infused} \times \text{dose} \times 60}{\text{amount of drug} \times 1,000}$$

where:

total volume to be infused = 500 mL

total amount of drug (mg) = 50 mg

dose = 10 mcg/min

60 converts minutes to hours

Substitute the numbers in the formula:

$$\frac{500 \times 10 \times 60}{50 \times 1,000} = 6\,mL/hour$$

Answer: The rate required = 6 mL/hour

Question 5   Lidocaine 0.2% in 500 mL at a rate of 2 mg/min

Before attempting the calculation, first estimate the required infusion rate.

Dose required = 2 mg/min – find the amount per hour (by multiplying by 60) = 2 × 60 = 120 mg/hour.

Next calculate the amount of lidocaine in the infusion.

Concentration is 0.2% which is equal to 0.2 g in 100 mL; for 500 mL, this equal to 0.2 × 5 = 1 g or 1,000 mg.

We have an infusion containing:

     1,000 mg   –   500 mL
     10 mg   –   5 mL   (by dividing by 100)
     120 mg   –   60 mL   (by multiplying by 12)

Infusion rate would be 60 mL/hour.

Although you have calculated the infusion rate required, it is always a good idea to do the calculation to check that you have the right answer.

Now we can attempt the calculation:

$$\text{Dose} = 2\ \text{mg/min}$$

The final answer is in terms of hours, so multiply by 60 to convert minutes into hours.

Dose = 2 mg/min = 2 × 60 = 120 mg/hour

Calculate the volume for 1 mg of drug.

You have: 0.2% which is 0.2 g in 100 mL; for 500 mL, this equal to 0.2 × 5 = 1 g or 1,000 mg:

$$1\,\text{mg} = \frac{500}{1{,}000} = 0.5\,\text{mL}$$

Thus for the dose of 120 mg, the volume is equal to:

$$120\ \text{mg} = 120 \times 0.5 = 60\ \text{mL/hour}$$

Checking the calculated answer of 60 mL/hour with our estimate of 60 mL/hour means that we should be confident that our calculated answer is correct.

Answer: The rate required = 60 mL/hour.

As the dose is being given as a total dose (not on a weight basis), the following formula is used:

$$\text{mL/hour} = \frac{\text{volume to be infused} \times \text{dose} \times 60}{\text{amount of drug}}$$

where:

total volume to be infused = 500 mL
total amount of drug (mg) = 1,000 mg
dose = 2 mg/min
60 converts minutes to hours

Substitute the numbers in the formula:

$$\frac{500 \times 2 \times 60}{1,000} = 60 \, \text{mL/hour}$$

Answer: The rate required = 60 mL/hour.

Question 6 Aminophylline 250 mg in 10 mL ampoules; reconstitute with 20 mL and administer as a 100 mL infusion over 60 min.

Dose = 0.5 mg/kg/hour over 12 hours; patient's weight = 63 kg.

Before attempting the calculation, first estimate the dose and the required infusion rate.

Dose required for the patient = 63 × 0.5 = 31.5 mg/hour (round down to 30 mg/hour).

Therefore for 12 hours, you will need 30 × 12 = 360 mg.

Looking at the numbers – 360 mg should be more than 10 mL (250 mg) and less than 20 mL (500 mg). The volume can be estimated by doing the following.

You have 250 mg in 10 mL – to make the calculation easier, round down to 240 mg (so both amounts are now in multiples of 12):

240 mg   –   10 mL
120 mg   –   5 mL   (by halving)
360 mg   –   15 mL   (multiplying by 3)

The volume to draw up should be approximately 15 mL.

Next calculate the infusion rate.

Infusion of 500 mL to be given over 12 hours (round down to 10 hours); hourly rate will be approximately:

$$\frac{500}{10} = 50 \, \text{mL/hour}$$

As the time of the infusion was rounded down, the actual rate should be slightly less – 45 mL/hour would be a good guess.

Now we can attempt the calculation:

Dose required for the patient = 63 × 0.5 = 31.5 mg/hour

Therefore for 12 hours, you will need 31.5 × 12 = 378 mg

You have 250 mg in 10 mL

Therefore 1 mg would equal $\dfrac{10}{250}$ mL (one unit rule).

Thus $378\,mg = \dfrac{10}{250} \times 378 = 15.12\,mL = 15mL$

rounded down.

Checking the calculated answer of 15 mL with our estimate of 15 mL means that we should be confident that our calculated answer is correct.

Answer: Add 15 mL (378 mg) to a 500 mL infusion bag.

As the infusion is to run over 12 hours, calculate the hourly rate.

500 mL to be given over 12 hours

Therefore hourly rate would equal 500/12 mL = 41.67 mL/hour = 41.7 mL/hour rounded up.

Checking the calculated answer of 41.7 mL/hour with our estimate of 45 mL/hour means that we should be confident that our calculated answer is correct.

Answer: 41.7 mL/hour

Question 7 Aciclovir is available as 500 mg vials – to be reconstituted with 20 mL Water for Injection. A 100 mL infusion should be given over 60 minutes.

Dose = 5 mg/kg every 8 hours. Patient's weight = 86 kg.

Before attempting the calculation, first estimate the answer.

Round up the weight to 90 kg

Dose required = 5 mg/kg; so 90 × 5 = 450 mg

We have aciclovir 500 mg – one vial will be sufficient which needs to be reconstituted with 20 mL.

Both the dose prescribed and the medicine on hand are in the same units.

The dose required of 450 mg is less than the strength of the medicine on hand – so the answer will be less than 20 mL.

We have: 500 mg – 20 mL
So: 50 mg – 2 mL   (dividing by 10)
It follows: 450 mg – 18 mL   (multiplying by 9)
Volume for dose = 18 mL (approx)

As the infusion is to run over 60 minutes, which is the same as 1 hour, then no further calculation is needed. Set the rate to 100 mL/hour.

Although we have calculated the dose and the rate needed, it is always a good idea to do the calculation to check that you have the right answer.

Now we can attempt the calculation:

First calculate the dose required:

$$5 \times 86 = 430 \text{ mg}$$

Next, calculate the volume of the reconstituted vial required:

$$500 \text{ mg} = 20 \text{ mL}$$

$$1 \text{ mg} = \frac{20}{500} \text{ mL}$$

Therefore for 430 mg:

$$430 \text{ mg} = \frac{20}{500} \times 430 = \frac{430}{25} = 17.2 \text{ mL} \text{ or } 17 \text{ mL rounded down}$$

Checking the calculated answer of 430 mg and 17 mL with our estimate of 450 mg and 18 mL means that we should be confident that our calculated answer is correct.

Answer: Add 17 mL (430 mg) to a 100 mL infusion bag.

As the infusion is to run over 60 minutes, which is the same as 1 hour, then no further calculation is needed. Set the rate to 100 mL/hour.

Answer: 100 mL/hour

Question 8   Glyceryl trinitrate 50 mg in 50 mL

Starting rate = 150 mcg/min. Infusion = 50 mg in 50 mL

Before attempting the calculation, first estimate the answer.

Dose = 150 mcg/min; multiply by 60 to convert minutes into hours

Dose = 150 mcg/min = 150 × 60 = 9,000 mcg/hour

The dose prescribed and the medicine on hand have different units and so a conversion is needed.

Convert from micrograms to milligrams.

Convert mcg to mg by dividing by 1,000:

$$\frac{9,000}{1,000} = 9 \, \text{mg/hour}$$

We have an infusion of 50 mg in 50 mL which is the same as 1 mg in 1 mL; so 9 mg/hour will be 9 mL/hour.

Although we have calculated the dose needed, it is always a good idea to do the calculation to check that you have the right answer.

Now we can attempt the calculation:

Dose = 150 mcg/min

The final answer is in terms of hours, so multiply by 60 to convert minutes into hours:

Dose = 150 mcg/min = 150 × 60 = 9,000 mcg/hour

Convert mcg to mg by dividing by 1,000:

$$\frac{9,000}{1,000} = 9 \, \text{mg/hour}$$

The next step is to calculate the volume for the dose required.

Calculate the volume for 1 mg of drug.

You have: 50 mg in 50 mL:

$$1 \, \text{mg} = \frac{50}{50} = 1 \, \text{mL}$$

Thus for the dose of 9 mg, the volume is equal to:

9 mg = 9 × 1 = 9 mL/hour

Checking the calculated answer of 9 mL/hour with our estimate of 9 mL/hour means that we should be confident that our calculated answer is correct.

Answer: The rate required = 9 mL/hour.

The dose is being given as a total dose (not on a weight basis), and the following formula is used:

$$\text{mL/hour} = \frac{\text{volume to be infused} \times \text{dose} \times 60}{\text{amount of drug} \times 1,000}$$

where:

total volume to be infused = 50 mL

total amount of drug (mg) = 50 mg

dose = 150 mcg/min

1,000 converts mcg to mg and 60 converts minutes to hours

Substitute the numbers in the formula:

$$\frac{50 \times 150 \times 60}{50 \times 1,000} = \frac{15 \times 6}{10} = \frac{90}{10} = 9 \text{ mL/hour}$$

Answer: The rate required = 9 mL/hour.

Question 9 Vancomycin 500 mg vials

Dose = 1 g and each vial needs to be diluted to 5 mg/mL

The rate of administration should not exceed 10 mg/min

Before attempting the calculation, first estimate the answer.

Each vial needs to be diluted with at least 100 mL

5 mg – 1 mL

500 mg – 100 mL (multiplying by 10)

So 1 g (2 × 500 mg) will need at least 200 mL – 250 mL is the nearest available infusion size.

Minimum rate = 10 mg/min; dose = 1 g

The dose prescribed and the medicine on hand have different units and so a conversion is needed. Convert from grams to milligrams.

Convert 1 g to milligrams; multiply by 1,000 – 1 g × 1,000 = 1,000 mg

Each 10 mg needs to be given over at least 1 min.

So for 1,000 mg, rate: 10 mg – 1 min

So 100 mg – 10 min (multiplying by 10)

It follows that 1,000 mg – 100 min (multiplying by 10).

So 250 mL needs to be given over at least 100 min; to convert to a rate in mL/hour:

Rate: 100 min – 250 mL

So 10 min – 25 mL (dividing by 10)

So 30 min – 75 mL (multiplying by 3)

It follows that 60 min – 150 mL (multiplying by 2)

Although we have calculated the rate needed, it is always a good idea to do the calculation to check that you have the right answer.

Now we can attempt the calculation:

Vancomycin 500 mg vials

Dose = 1 g and each vial needs to be diluted to 5 mg/mL

The rate of administration should not exceed 10 mg/min

You need a final concentration of 5 mg/mL which is the same as:

$$\frac{1}{5} \text{ mg} = 1 \text{ mL}$$

The dose prescribed and the medicine on hand have different units and so a conversion is needed. Convert from grams to milligrams.

Convert 1 g to milligrams; multiply by 1,000, so 1 g × 1,000 = 1,000 mg

A dose of 1 g (1,000 mg) would need:

$$\frac{1}{5} \times 1,000 = 200 \text{ mL}$$

So 1 g (2 × 500 mg) will need at least 200 mL, so 250 mL is the nearest available infusion size.

Checking the calculated answer of 250 mL with our estimate of 250 mL means that we should be confident that our calculated answer is correct.
Answer: 250 mL

Maximum rate is 10 mg/minute, i.e. for every minute give 10 mg vancomycin.

So 1 mg needs to be given over at least: $\frac{1}{10}$ minutes.

For a dose of 1 g or 1,000 mg: $\frac{1}{10} \times 1,000 = 100$ minutes.

Checking the calculated answer of 100 min with our estimate of 100 min means that we should be confident that our calculated answer is correct.
Answer: 100 minutes

Need to give 250 mL fluid over 100 minutes.

As the pump needs to be set as per hour, we need to calculate the volume to be given over 60 minutes:

$$1 \text{ minute} = \frac{250}{100} \text{ mL}$$

$$60 \text{ minutes} = \frac{250}{100} \times 60 = 150 \text{ mL/hour}$$

Checking the calculated answer of 150 mL/hour with our estimate of 150 mL/hour means that we should be confident that our calculated answer is correct.
Answer: 150 mL/hour

Question 10   Dobutamine 250 mg in 500 mL

Patient's weight = 73 kg; dose = 5 mcg/kg/min

Before attempting the calculation, first estimate the answer.

Round up the weight to 75 kg.

Dose = 75 × 5 = 375 mcg/min

As the weight has been rounded up, then the actual answer should be slightly lower, so 370 mcg/min would be a good guess.

We have 250 mg in 500 mL

Find the amount in 1 mL and then convert to micrograms:

We have:	500 mL – 250 mg	
So:	50 mL – 25 mg	(dividing by 10)
So:	10 mL – 5 mg	(dividing by 5)
It follows:	1 mL – 0.5 mg	(dividing by 10)

The dose prescribed and the medicine on hand have different units and so a conversion is needed. Convert from milligrams to micrograms.

Converting milligrams to micrograms, multiply by 1,000:

$$0.5 \text{ mg} \times 1,000 = 500 \text{ micrograms/mL}$$

To find the rate in mL/hour, convert the amount per minute to an amount per hour and then convert that amount to a volume.

To make calculations easier, split the calculation into two parts.

We have 375 mcg/min; multiply by 60 (multiply by 6 then by 10):

$$375 \times 6 = 2,250 \times 10 = 22,500 \text{ micrograms/hour}$$

We know that the infusion contains 500 micrograms in 1 mL.

We have:	500 mcg – 1 mL	
So:	1,000 mcg – 2 mL	(multiplying by 2)
So:	2,000 mcg – 4 mL	(multiplying by 2)
So:	20,000 mcg – 40 mL	(multiplying by 10)

It follows:	20,000 mcg	– 40 mL
	2,000 mcg	– 4 mL
	+ 500 mcg	– +1 mL
	22,500 mcg	45 mL

Rate = 45 mL/hour

(By addition; 20,000 mcg + 2,000 mcg + 500 mcg or 40 mL + 4 mL + 1 mL)

As the dose has been rounded up, the actual answer should be slightly lower – 43 mL/hour would be a good guess.

Although we have calculated the rate needed, it is always a good idea to do the calculation to check that you have the right answer.

Now we can attempt the calculation:

First calculate the dose required:

$$\text{dose required} = \text{patient's weight} \times \text{dose prescribed}$$
$$= 73 \times 5 = 365 \text{ mcg/min}$$

Checking the calculated answer of 365 mcg/min with our estimate of 370 mcg/min means that we should be confident that our calculated answer is correct.

Answer: 365 mcg/min

You have 250 mg in 500 mL:

$$1 \text{ mL} = \frac{250}{500} = 0.5 \text{ mg}$$

The dose prescribed and the medicine on hand have different units and so a conversion is needed.

Converting milligrams to micrograms, multiply by 1,000:

$$0.5 \text{ mg} \times 1,000 = 500 \text{ micrograms/mL}$$

Checking the calculated answer of 500 mcg/mL with our estimate of 500 mcg/mL means that we should be confident that our calculated answer is correct.

Answer: 0.5 mg/mL or 500 mcg/mL

Dose = 365 mcg/min. The final answer is in terms of hours, so multiply by 60 to convert minutes into hours.

Dose = 365 mcg/min = 365×60 = 21,900 mcg/hour

Convert mcg to mg by dividing by 1,000:
$$\frac{21,900}{1,000} = 21.9 \text{ mg/hour}.$$

The next step is to calculate the volume for the dose required.

Calculate the volume for 1 mg of drug.

You have: 250 mg in 500 mL

$$1 \text{ mg} = \frac{500}{250} = 2 \text{ mL}$$

Thus for the dose of 21.9 mg, the volume is equal to: 21.9 × 2 = 43.8 mL/hour.

Checking the calculated answer of 43.8 mL/hour with our estimate of 43 mL/hour means that we should be confident that our calculated answer is correct.

Answer: The rate required = 43.8 mL/hour

Question 11   Infusion of isosorbide dinitrate 50 mg in 500 mL at a rate of 2 mg/hour

Before attempting the calculation, first estimate the answer.

Convert the amount to a volume, for 2 mg/hour.

We have: 50 mg – 500 mL

So: 1 mg – 10 mL   (dividing by 50)

It follows: 2 mg – 20 mL   (multiplying by 2)

Rate = 20 mL/hour

Although we have calculated the answer needed, it is always a good idea to do the calculation to check that you have the right answer.

Now we can attempt the calculation:

The rate = 2 mg/hour, convert mg to mL

You have 50 mg in 500 mL

$$\text{Therefore } 1 \text{ mg} = \frac{500}{50} = 10 \text{ mL}$$

Thus 2 mg/hour = 10 × 2 = 20 mL/hour

Checking the calculated answer of 20 mL/hour with our estimate of 20 mL/hour means that we should be confident that our calculated answer is correct.

Answer: The rate = 20 mL/hour

The rate is now changed to 5 mg/hour.

Before attempting the calculation, first estimate the answer.

Convert the amount to a volume, for 5 mg/hour.

We have: 50 mg – 500 mL

So: 1 mg – 10 mL   (dividing by 50)

It follows: 5 mg – 50 mL   (multiplying by 5)

Although we have calculated the answer needed, it is always a good idea to do the calculation to check that you have the right answer.

Now we can attempt the calculation:

The new rate = 5 mg/hour which is equal to 10 × 5 = 50 mL/hour (as 1 mg = 10 mL; calculated before).

Checking the calculated answer of 50 mL/hour with our estimate of 50 mL/hour means that we should be confident that our calculated answer is correct.

Answer: The rate = 50 mL/hour

Question 12 Dopamine 800 mg in 500 mL and the initial dose required is 2 mcg/kg/min and increased in increments of 1 mcg to a maximum of 5 mcg/kg/min. Patient's weight is 80 kg.

Before attempting the calculation, first estimate the answer.

Maintain the weight at 80 kg.

So for a unit dose = 1 mcg/min × 80 kg = 80 mcg/min

Multiply by 60 to convert to hours:

$$80 \times 60 = 4{,}800 \text{ mcg/hour}$$

The dose prescribed and the medicine on hand have different units and so a conversion is needed.

Convert micrograms to milligrams by dividing by 1,000:

$$\frac{4{,}800}{1{,}000} = 4.8 \text{ mg/hour}$$

For ease of calculation, round up the rate to 5 mg/hour.

We have:	800 mg – 500 mL	
So:	400 mg – 250 mL	(by halving)
So:	100 mg – 62.5 mL	(dividing by 4)
So:	50 mg – 31.25 mL	(by halving)
It follows:	5 mg – 3.125 mL	(dividing by 10)

As the rate has been rounded up, then the actual answer should be less than the estimated answer – around 3.1 mL/hour would be a good guess.

Now we can attempt the calculation:

First calculate the dose required for a unit dose of 1 mcg/kg/min:

$$\text{dose required} = \text{patient's weight} \times \text{unit dose}$$
$$= 80 \times 1 = 80 \text{ mcg/min}$$

Dose = 80 mcg/min. The final answer is in terms of hours, so multiply by 60 to convert minutes into hours:

dose = 80 mcg/min = 80 × 60 = 4,800 mcg/hour

The dose prescribed and the medicine on hand have different units and so a conversion is needed.

Convert micrograms to milligrams by dividing by 1,000:

$$\frac{4,800}{1,000} = 4.8 \, mg/hour$$

The next step is to calculate the volume for the dose required.

Calculate the volume for 1 mg of drug.

You have: 800 mg in 500 mL:

$$1 \, mg = \frac{500}{800} = 0.625 \, mL$$

Thus for the unit dose of 4.8 mg, the volume is equal to: 4.8 × 0.625 = 3 (there is no need to round up to one decimal place = 3 mL/hour).

Checking the calculated answer of 3 mL/hour with our estimate of 3.1 mL/hour means that we should be confident that our calculated answer is correct.

Next calculate the rate for each incremental step.

Answer: 2 mcg/kg/min = 6 mL/hour
3 mcg/kg/min = 9 mL/hour
4 mcg/kg/min = 12 mL/hour
5 mcg/kg/min = 15 mL/hour

Using the formula to calculate the unit dose:

$$mL/hour = \frac{volume \ to \ be \ infused \times dose \times wgt \times 60}{amount \ of \ drug \times 1,000}$$

In this case:

Total volume to be infused = 500 mL
Total amount of drug (mg) = 800 mg
Dose   = 1 mcg/kg/min
Patient's weight (wgt)   = 80 kg
60 converts minutes to hours
1,000 converts mcg to mg

Substitute the numbers in the formula:

$$\frac{500 \times 1 \times 80 \times 60}{800 \times 1,000} = 3 \text{ mL/hour}$$

Next calculate the rate for each incremental step.
Answer: 2 mcg/kg/min = 6 mL/hour
3 mcg/kg/min = 9 mL/hour
4 mcg/kg/min = 12 mL/hour
5 mcg/kg/min = 15 mL/hour

Question 13 Dobutamine 250 mg in 50 mL and the initial dose required is 2.5 mcg/kg/min and increased in increments of 2.5 mcg to a maximum of 10 mcg/kg/min. Patient's weight is 75 kg.

Before attempting the calculation, first estimate the answer.

Maintain the weight at 75 kg.

So for a unit dose = 1 mcg/min × 75 kg = 75 mcg/min

Multiply by 60 to convert to hours:

$$75 \times 60 = 4,500 \text{ mcg/hour}$$

The dose prescribed and the medicine on hand have different units and so a conversion is needed.

Convert micrograms to milligrams by dividing by 1,000:

$$\frac{4,500}{1,000} = 4.5 \text{ mg/hour}$$

For ease of calculation, round up the rate to 5 mg/hour.

We have: 250 mg – 50 mL
So: 50 mg – 10 mL (dividing by 5)
It follows: 5 mg – 1 mL (dividing by 10)

As the rate has been rounded up, then the actual answer should be less than the estimated answer – around 0.9 mL/hour would be a good guess.

Now we can attempt the calculation:

First calculate the dose required for a unit dose of 1 mcg/kg/min:

dose required = patient's weight × unit dose
= 75 × 1 = 75 mcg/min

Dose = 75 mcg/min. The final answer is in terms of hours, so multiply by 60 to convert minutes into hours:

dose = 75 mcg/min = 75 × 60 = 4,500 mcg/hour

Convert mcg to mg by dividing by 1,000: $\dfrac{4,500}{1,000}$ = 4.5 mg/hour

The next step is to calculate the volume for the dose required.

Calculate the volume for 1 mg of drug.

You have: 250 mg in 50 mL:

$$1\,mg\ \dfrac{50}{250} = 0.2\,mL$$

Thus for the unit dose of 4.5 mg, the volume is equal to: 4.5 × 0.2 = 0.9 (round up to one decimal place = 0.9 mL/hour).

Checking the calculated answer of 0.9 mL/hour with our estimate of 0.9 mL/hour means that we should be confident that our calculated answer is correct.

Next calculate the rate for each incremental step:

1 mcg/kg/min = 0.9 mL/hour
2.5 mcg/kg/min = 2.5 × 0.9 = 2.25 mL/hour
(round up to one decimal place = 2.3 mL/hour)

Answer: 2.5 mcg/kg/min = 2.3 mL/hour
5 mcg/kg/min   = 4.6 mL/hour
7.5 mcg/kg/min = 6.9 mL/hour
10 mcg/kg/min = 9.2 mL/hour

Using the formula to calculate the unit dose:

$$mL/hour\ =\ \dfrac{volume\ to\ be\ infused\ \times\ dose\ \times\ wgt\ \times\ 60}{amount\ of\ drug\ \times\ 1,000}$$

In this case: total volume to be infused = 250 mL
Total amount of drug (mg)   = 50 mg
Dose   = 1 mcg/kg/min
Patient's weight (wgt)   = 75 kg
60 converts minutes to hours and 1,000 converts mcg to mg

Substitute the numbers in the formula:

$$\frac{50 \times 1 \times 75 \times 60}{250 \times 1,000} = 0.9 \text{ mL/hour}$$

Next calculate the rate for each incremental step:

1 mcg/kg/min = 0.9 mL/hour
2.5 mcg/kg/min = 2.5 × 0.9 = 2.25 mL/hour
(round up to one decimal place = 2.3 mL/hour)

Answer: 2.5 mcg/kg/min = 2.3 mL/hour
5 mcg/kg/min   = 4.6 mL/hour
7.5 mcg/kg/min = 6.9 mL/hour
10 mcg/kg/min = 9.2 mL/hour

Conversion of mL/hour to dosages

Question 14   Dopamine 200 mg in 50 mL and the rate = 4 mL/hour

The prescribed dose is 3 mcg/kg/min and patient's weight = 89 kg

Before attempting the calculation, first estimate the original dose. Don't forget, this is only an estimate – it will only detect large discrepancies, not small ones such as less than 0.5 mL.

The current rate is 4 mL/hour.

Next, we need to convert the volume to an amount.

We have:	50 mL – 200 mg	
So:	10 mL – 40 mg	(dividing by 5)
So:	1 mL – 4 mg	(dividing by 10)
It follows:	4 mL – 16 mg	(multiplying by 4)

The rate can be rewritten as 16 mg/hour

The dose prescribed and the rate have different units and so a conversion is needed. Convert milligrams to micrograms – multiply by 1,000.

So, 16 × 1,000 = 16,000 mcg/hour

Next convert to an amount per minute. For ease of calculation, round up the dose to 18,000 mcg/hour:

We have:	18,000 mcg – 60 min	
So:	9,000 mcg – 30 min	(dividing by 2)
So:	3,000 mcg – 10 min	(dividing by 3)
It follows:	300 mcg – 1 min	(dividing by 10)

To calculate the dose, the weight needs to be taken into account: weight = 89 kg – round up to 90 kg. To find the dose, divide by the weight:

$$\frac{300}{90} = \frac{30}{9} = \frac{10}{3} = 3.33 \text{ mcg/kg/min}$$

As the rate has been rounded up, the actual dose will be slightly less – 3 mcg/kg/min would be a good guess.

It has been estimated that the dose is correct and no adjustment is necessary.

Although we have calculated the answer needed, it is always a good idea to do the calculation to check that you have the right answer.

Now we can attempt the calculation:

You have 200 mg of dopamine in 50 mL

First calculate the amount in 1 mL

You have 200 mg in 50 mL

Therefore $1 \text{ mL} = \frac{200}{50} \text{ mg} = 4 \text{ mg}$ (using the one unit rule)

The rate at which the pump is running is 4 mL/hour, therefore for 4 mL:

$$4 \text{ mL/hour} = 4 \times 4 = 16 \text{ mg/hour}$$

Convert milligrams to micrograms by multiplying by 1,000:

$$16 \times 1,000 = 16,000 \text{ mcg/hour}$$

Now calculate the rate per minute by dividing by 60 (converts hours to minutes):

$$\frac{16,000}{60} = 266.67 \text{ mcg/min}$$

The final step in the calculation is to work out the rate according to the patient's weight (89 kg):

$$\frac{266.67}{89} = 2.996 \text{ mcg/kg/min} = 3 \text{ mcg/kg/min}$$

Checking the calculated answer of 3 mcg/kg/min with our estimate of 3 mcg/kg/min means that we should be confident that our calculated answer is correct.

Answer: The dose is correct. No adjustment is necessary. Using the formula:

$$\text{mcg/kg/hour} = \frac{\text{rate (mL/hour)} \times \text{amount of drug} \times 1,000}{\text{weight (kg)} \times \text{volume (mL)} \times 60}$$

where in this case:

rate	= 4 mL/hour
amount of drug (mg)	= 200 mg
weight (kg)	= 89 kg
volume (mL)	= 50 mL

60 converts minutes to hours and 1,000 converts mg to mcg.

Substitute the numbers in the formula:

$$\frac{4 \times 200 \times 1,000}{89 \times 50 \times 60} = 2.99 \text{ mcg/kg/min} = 3 \text{ mcg/kg/min}$$

Answer: The dose is correct. No adjustment is necessary.

Question 15   Dobutamine 250 mg in 50 mL and the rate = 5.4 mL/hour

The prescribed dose is 6 mcg/kg/min and patient's weight = 64 kg.

Before attempting the calculation, first estimate the original dose. Don't forget, this is only an estimate – it will only detect large discrepancies, not small ones such as less than 0.5 mL.

The current rate is 5.4 mL/hour.

Next, we need to convert the volume to an amount.

We have:	50 mL – 250 mg	
So:	5 mL – 25 mg	(dividing by 10)
So:	1 mL – 5 mg	(dividing by 5)
So:	0.2 mL – 1 mg	(dividing by 5)
So:	0.4 mL – 2 mg	(multiplying by 2)
It follows:	5.4 mL – 27 mg	(by addition: 5 mL + 0.4 mL or 25 mg + 2 mg)

The rate can be rewritten as 27 mg/hour.

Next convert to an amount per minute:

We have:	27 mg – 60 min	
So:	9 mg – 20 min	(dividing by 3)
So:	4.5 mg – 10 min	(dividing by 2)
It follows:	0.45 mg – 1 min	(dividing by 10)

As the dose is given in micrograms, convert the above to micrograms:

$$0.45 \text{ mg/min} = 0.45 \times 1,000 = 450 \text{ mcg/min}$$

So 27 × 1,000 = 27,000 mcg/hour.

To calculate the dose, the weight needs to be taken into account: weight = 64 kg – round up to 65 kg. To find the dose, divide by the weight:

$$\frac{450}{65} = \frac{90}{13} \text{ which is approximately } \frac{91}{13} = 7 \text{ mcg/kg/min}$$

Dose = 7 mcg/kg/min

It has been estimated that the dose is incorrect and some adjustment is necessary.

Although we have calculated the answer needed, it is always a good idea to do the calculation to check that you have the right answer. You may have noticed that the estimation method used is different to that for the last question. It illustrates that more than one method can be used.

Now we can attempt the calculation:

We have 250 mg of dobutamine in 50 mL

First calculate the amount in 1 mL

You have 250 mg in 50 mL

Therefore $1 \text{ mL} = \dfrac{200}{50} \text{ mg} = 5 \text{ mg}$ (using the one unit rule).

The rate at which the pump is running is 5.4 mL/hour, therefore for 5.4 mL:

$$5.4 \text{ mL/hour} = 5.4 \times 5 = 27 \text{ mg/hour}$$

Convert milligrams to micrograms by multiplying by 1,000:

$$27 \times 1,000 = 27,000 \text{ mcg/hour}$$

Now calculate the rate per minute by dividing by 60 (converts hours to minutes):

$$\frac{27,000}{60} = 450 \text{ mcg/min}$$

Next work out the rate according to the patient's weight (64 kg):

$$\frac{450}{64} = 7.03 \text{ mcg/kg/min (7 mcg/kg/min, rounded down)}$$

Checking the calculated answer of 7 mcg/kg/min with our estimate of 7 mcg/kg/min means that we should be confident that our calculated answer is correct.

Answer: 7.03 mcg/kg/min (7 mcg/kg/min, rounded down)

The dose being delivered by the pump set at a rate of 5.4 mL/hour is too high. Inform the doctor and adjust the rate of the pump.

Using the formula:

$$\text{mcg/kg/min} = \frac{\text{rate (mL/hour)} \times \text{amount of drug} \times 1,000}{\text{weight (kg)} \times \text{volume (mL)} \times 60}$$

where in this case:

rate	=	5.4 mL/hour
amount of drug (mg)	=	250 mg
weight (kg)	=	64 kg
volume (mL)	=	50 mL

60 converts minutes to hours and 1,000 converts mg to mcg.

Substitute the numbers in the formula:

$$\frac{5.4 \times 250 \times 1,000}{64 \times 50 \times 60} = 7.03 \text{ mcg/kg/min (7 mcg/kg/min)}$$

Answer: 7.03 mcg/kg/min (7 mcg/kg/min, rounded down)

The dose being delivered by the pump set at a rate of 5.4 mL/hour is too high. Inform the doctor and adjust the rate of the pump.

Changing the rate of the pump

Before attempting the calculation, first estimate the answer.

In this case, the calculation is done the other way – starting at the dose.

First calculate the dose required:

$$\text{dose required} = \text{patient's weight} \times \text{dose prescribed}$$
$$= 64 \times 6 = 384 \text{ mcg/min}$$

Dose = 384 mcg/min. The final answer is in terms of hours, so multiply by 60 to convert minutes into hours.

To make the calculation easier, multiply by 6 and then by 10:

dose = 384 mcg/min = 384 × 6 = 2,304 × 10
= 23,040 mcg/hour

Once again, to make the calculation easier, round down the dose to 23,000 mcg/hour.

The dose prescribed and the medicine on hand have different units and so a conversion is needed.

Convert from micrograms to milligrams.

Convert mcg to mg by dividing by 1,000:

$$\frac{23,000}{1,000} = 23\,mg/hour.$$

We have:	250 mg of dobutamine in 50 mL	
We have:	250 mg – 50 mL	
So:	10 mg – 2 mL	(dividing by 25)
So:	20 mg – 4 mL	(multiplying by 2)
So:	1 mg – 0.2 mL	(dividing by 20)
So:	3 mg – 0.6 mL	(multiplying by 3)
It follows:	23 mg – 4.6 mL	(by addition; 20 mg + 3 mg or 4 mL + 0.6 mL)

The rate can be rewritten as 4.6 mL/hour

Although we have calculated the answer needed, it is always a good idea to do the calculation to check that you have the right answer.

Now we can attempt the calculation.

Changing the rate of the pump

In this case, the calculation is done the other way round – starting at the dose.

First calculate the dose required:

dose required = patient's weight × dose prescribed
= 64 × 6 = 384 mcg/min

Dose = 384 mcg/min. The final answer is in terms of hours, so multiply by 60 to convert minutes into hours:

dose = 384 mcg/min = 384 × 60 = 23,040 mcg/hour

Convert mcg to mg by dividing by 1,000:

$$\frac{23,040}{1,000} = 23.04\,mg/hour.$$

The next step is to calculate the volume for the dose required.

Calculate the volume for 1 mg of drug.

You have: 250 mg in 50 mL

Therefore $1\,mg = \dfrac{50}{250} = 0.2\,mL$

Thus for the dose of 23.04 mg, the volume is equal to:

$$23.04\ mg = 23.04 \times 0.2 = 4.608\ mL/hour$$
$$(4.6\ mL/hour,\ rounded\ to\ one\ decimal\ place)$$

Checking the calculated answer of 4.6 mL/hour with our estimate of 4.6 mL/hour means that we should be confident that our calculated answer is correct.

Answer: The rate at which the pump should have been set equals 4.6 mL/hour and not 5.4 mL/hour.

A formula can be devised:

$$mL/hour = \frac{volume\ to\ be\ infused \times dose \times wgt \times 60}{amount\ of\ drug \times 1{,}000}$$

where in this case:

total volume to be infused	=	50 mL
total amount of drug (mg)	=	250 mg
dose	=	6 mcg/kg/min
patient's weight (wgt)	=	64 kg

60 converts minutes to hours and 1,000 converts mcg to mg

Substitute the numbers in the formula:

$$\frac{50 \times 6 \times 64 \times 60}{250 \times 1{,}000} = 4.608\ mL/hour\ (4.6\ mL/hour,\ approx.)$$

Answer: The rate at which the pump should have been set equals 4.6 mL/hour and not 5.4 mL/hour.

Question 16 Dopexamine 50 mg in 50 mL and the rate = 28 mL/hour

The prescribed dose is 6 mcg/kg/min. Patient's weight = 78 kg.

Before attempting the calculation, first estimate the original dose. Don't forget, this is only an estimate – it will only detect large discrepancies, not small ones such as less than 0.5 mL.

The current rate is 28 mL/hour and we need to convert the volume to an amount. We have 50 mg in

50 mL which is the same as 1 mg in 1 mL; so 28 mL = 28 mg.

The rate can be rewritten as 28 mg/hour.

The dose prescribed and the rate have different units and so a conversion is needed. Convert milligrams to micrograms – multiply by 1,000.

So 28 × 1,000 = 28,000 mcg/hour

Next convert to an amount per minute. For ease of calculation, round up the dose to 30,000 mcg/hour.

We have: 30,000 mcg – 60 min

So: 1,000 mcg – 2 min (dividing by 30)

It follows: 500 mcg – 1 min (dividing by 2)

To calculate the dose, the weight needs to be taken into account; weight = 78 kg – round up to 80 kg. To find the dose, divide by the weight:

$$\frac{500}{80} = \frac{50}{8} \text{ which is approximately } \frac{48}{8} = 6 \text{ mcg/kg/min}$$

Our estimation indicates that the pump is set at the correct rate as it is delivering a dose of 6 mcg/kg/min.

Although we have calculated the answer needed, it is always a good idea to do the calculation to check that you have the right answer.

Now we can attempt the calculation:

You have 50 mg of dopexamine in 50 mL

First calculate the amount in 1 mL

You have 50 mg in 50 mL

Therefore $1 \text{ mL} = \frac{50}{50} \text{ mg} = 1\text{mg}$ (using the one unit rule)

The rate at which the pump is running is 28 mL/hour, therefore for 28 mL:

$$28 \text{ mL/hour} = 28 \times 1 = 28 \text{ mg/hour}$$

The dose prescribed and the rate have different units and so a conversion is needed. Convert milligrams to micrograms – multiply by 1,000.

So 28 × 1,000 = 28,000 mcg/hour.

Now calculate the rate per minute by dividing by 60 (converts hours to minutes):

$$\frac{28,000}{60} = 466.67 \text{ mcg/min}$$

The final step in the calculation is to work out the rate according to the patient's weight (78 kg):

$$\frac{466.67}{78} = 5.98 \text{ mcg/kg/min} = 6 \text{ mcg/kg/min, rounded up)}$$

Checking the calculated answer of 6 mcg/kg/min with our estimate of 6 mcg/kg/min means that we should be confident that our calculated answer is correct.

Answer: The dose is correct. No adjustment is necessary.

Using the formula:

$$\text{mcg/kg/min} = \frac{\text{rate (mL/hour)} \times \text{amount of drug} \times 1{,}000}{\text{weight (kg)} \times \text{volume (mL)} \times 60}$$

where in this case:

rate	=	28 mL/hour
amount of drug (mg)	=	50 mg
weight (kg)	=	78 kg
volume (mL)	=	50 mL

60 converts minutes to hours and 1,000 converts mg to mcg.

Substitute the numbers in the formula:

$$\frac{28 \times 50 \times 1{,}000}{78 \times 50 \times 60} = 5.98 \text{ mcg/kg/min}$$
$$= 6 \text{ mcg/kg/min, rounded up}$$

Answer: The dose is correct. No adjustment is necessary.

Calculating the length of time for IV infusion

Question 17   Infusion = 500 mL being given over 4 hours

Standard giving set at a rate of 42 drops/min

Before attempting the calculation, first estimate the length of time for the infusion. In this case, convert drops to a volume and minutes to hours.

To make calculations easier, round down the drip rate to 40 drops/min.

We know that 20 drops equals to 1 mL; so 40 drops would equal to 2 mL.

Next, calculate the time taken to administer 500 mL.

We have: 2 mL – 1 min
So: 100 mL – 50 min   (multiplying by 50)
It follows: 500 mL – 250 min   (multiplying by 5)

Finally, convert minutes to hours by dividing by 60:

$$\frac{250}{60} = \frac{25}{6} \text{ which is approximately } \frac{24}{6} = 4 \text{ hours}$$

Although we have calculated the answer needed, it is always a good idea to do the calculation to check that you have the right answer.

Now we can attempt the calculation:

First, convert the volume to drops by multiplying the volume of the infusion by the number of drops/mL for the giving set:

$$500 \times 20 = 10,000 \text{ drops}$$

Next, calculate how many minutes it will take for 1 drop, i.e.

$$42 \text{ drops per minute}$$

$$1 \text{ drop} = \frac{1}{42} \text{ min}$$

Calculate how many minutes it will take to infuse the total number of drops:

$$10,000 \text{ drops } \frac{1}{42} \times 10,000 = 238 \text{ min}$$

Convert minutes to hours by dividing by 60:

$$238 \text{ mins} = \frac{238}{60} = 3.97 \text{ hours}$$

$$3.97 \text{ hours} = 3 \text{ hours } 58 \text{ min (approx. 4 hours)}$$

Checking the calculated answer of 4 hours with our estimate of 4 hours means that we should be confident that our calculated answer is correct.

Answer: 500 mL of sodium chloride 0.9% at a rate of 42 drops/min will take approximately 4 hours to run.

If using the formula:

$$\frac{\text{number of hours the}}{\text{infusion is to run}} = \frac{\text{volume of the infusion}}{\text{rate (drops/min)} \times 60} \times \frac{\text{drip rate of}}{\text{giving set}}$$

where:

volume of the infusion	=	500 mL
rate (drops/min)	=	42 drops/min
drip rate of giving set	=	20 drops/mL

Substitute the numbers in the formula:

$$\frac{500 \times 20}{42 \times 60} = 3.97 \text{ hours}$$

3.97 hours = 3 hours 58 min (approx. 4 hours)

Answer: 500 mL of sodium chloride 0.9% at a rate of 42 drops/min will take approximately 4 hours to run.

Question 18 Infusion = 1 litre being given over 12 hours

Rate = 83 mL/hour

Before attempting the calculation, first estimate the length of time for the infusion.

To make calculations easier, round down the rate to 80 mL/hour.

The infusion and the rate have different units and so a conversion is needed. Convert litres to millilitres – multiply by 1,000:

$$1 \times 1,000 = 1,000 \text{ mL}$$

We have: 80 mL – 1 hour

So: 40 mL – 0.5 hours (by halving)

So: 200 mL – 2.5 hours (by multiplying by 5)

It follows: 1,000 mL – 12.5 hours (by multiplying by 5)

As the rate has been rounded down, then the actual answer should be slightly lower – 12 hours would be a good guess.

Although we have calculated the answer needed, it is always a good idea to do the calculation to check that you have the right answer.

Now we can attempt the calculation:

Divide the volume by the rate to give you the time over which the infusion is to run.

Calculated rate = 83 mL/hour

Volume = 1,000 mL

$$\frac{1,000}{83} = 12.05 \text{ hours (12 hours approx.)}$$

Checking the calculated answer of 12 hours with our estimate of 12 hours means that we should be confident that our calculated answer is correct.

Answer: 1 litre of sodium chloride 0.9% at a rate of 83 mL/hour will take 12 hours to run.

Using the formula:

$$\frac{\text{number of hours the}}{\text{infusion is to run}} = \frac{\text{volume of the infusion}}{\text{rate (mL/hour)}}$$

where in this case:

volume of the infusion = 1,000 mL
rate (mL/hour)   = 83 mL/hour

Substitute the numbers in the formula:

$$\frac{1,000}{83} = 12.05 \text{ hours (12 hours approx.)}$$

Answer: 1 litre of sodium chloride 0.9% at a rate of 83 mL/hour will take 12 hours to run.

Chapter 10 Action and administration of medicines

Question 1   Answer: 0.37 mL
Question 2   Answer: 0.83 mL
Question 3   Answer: 0.56 mL
Question 4   Answer: 0.75 mL
Question 5   Answer: 1.4 mL
Question 6   Answer: 1.8 mL
Question 7   Answer: 2.8 mL
Question 8   Answer: 3.6 mL
Question 9   Answer: 6.5 mL
Question 10   Answer: 8.0 mL

Appendices

Appendix I

BODY SURFACE AREA (BSA) ESTIMATES

Many physiological phenomena correlate to body surface area (BSA) and for this reason some drugs are calculated using BSA.

Cancer chemotherapy is usually dosed using BSA. BSA has been chosen rather than body weight to calculate doses for two reasons:

- It provides a more accurate estimation of effect and toxicity.
- It more closely correlates to blood flow to the liver and kidneys, which are the major organs for drug elimination.

Cancer drugs have a lower therapeutic index (the difference between an effective and a toxic dose) than most other drugs, i.e. the difference between an underdose and an overdose is small and the consequences can be life threatening. Therefore, cancer chemotherapy needs a precise and reliable method of determining the BSA and dose.

Paediatric doses can be estimated more accurately using BSA, and some drugs (e.g. aciclovir) have doses based on BSA.

Several different formulae and nomograms have been derived for predicting surface area from measurements of height and weight. For accuracy, BSA should be calculated to three significant figures. Slide rules and nomograms are incapable of calculating with this degree of accuracy. In addition, they suffer from error associated with their analogue nature and the formulae on which they are based.

FORMULAE FOR CALCULATING BODY SURFACE AREA

There are many formulae for calculating BSA. The formula derived by Mosteller (1987) combines an accurate BSA calculation with ease of use and has been validated for use in both children and adults. This formula can be used on a handheld calculator.

Mosteller formula:

$$m^2 = \sqrt{\frac{\text{Height}\,(\text{cm}) \times \text{Weight}\,(\text{kg})}{3600}}$$

For example, you want to know the BSA of a child whose weight is 16.4 kg and height 100 cm.

Substitute the figures in the formula:

$$m^2 = \sqrt{\frac{100 \times 16.4}{3600}}$$

$$m^2 = \sqrt{\frac{1640}{3600}}$$

$$m^2 = \sqrt{0.456} = 0.675$$

First, do the sum in the top line: $100 \times 16.4 = 1640$.
Next, divide by 3,600 to give 0.456.
Finally, find the square root to give an answer of 0.675.

ONLINE CALCULATORS

In 1916, Du Bois and Du Bois derived a formula to estimate BSA on which many nomograms are based. Although they used measurements of only nine individuals, one of whom was a child, and made certain assumptions in developing the formula, this remains the most popular online calculator for calculating BSA.

The Mosteller BSA calculator can be found at: http://www.patient.co.uk/doctor/body-surface-area-calculator-mosteller

The DuBois BSA calculator can be found at: https://www.medicinescomplete.com/mc/bnf/current/PHP18585-body-surface-area.htm

Reference

Mosteller RD. Simplified calculation of body-surface area. *N Engl J Med* 1987; 317:1098.

Appendix 2

WEIGHT CONVERSION TABLES

Although conversion charts exist, these may not always be at hand, so knowing how to convert is helpful. Sometimes it may be necessary to convert stones and pounds to kilograms and vice versa. Patients' weights are usually given in stones and have to be converted to kilograms, especially when working out dosages. A lot of dosages are calculated on a 'weight basis', e.g. mg/kg/day.

There are many calculators and converters available on the Internet. The British National Formulary (BNF) on-line converter can be accessed at: https://www.medicinescomplete.com/mc/bnf/current/PHP18592-weight.htm

The following table shows weight conversions.

STONES TO KILOGRAMS		POUNDS TO KILOGRAMS	
STONES	KILOGRAMS	POUNDS	KILOGRAMS
1	6.4	1	0.5
2	12.7	2	0.9
3	19.1	3	1.4
4	25.4	4	1.8
5	31.8	5	2.3
6	38.1	6	2.7
7	44.5	7	3.2
8	50.8	8	3.6
9	57.2	9	4.1
10	63.5	10	4.5
11	69.9	11	5.0
12	76.2	12	5.4
13	82.6	13	5.9
14	88.9		
15	95.3		
16	101.6		
17	108.0		
18	114.3		
19	120.7		
20	127.0		
21	133.4		

Note: Weights in kg correct to 0.1 kg.

Conversion factors are as follows:
Stones to kilograms $\times$ 6.3503
Pounds to kilograms $\times$ 0.4536
Kilograms to stones $\times$ 0.1575
Kilograms to pounds $\times$ 2.2046

WORKED EXAMPLE

Convert 14 stones 4 pounds to kilograms (to the nearest kg).

Using the conversion table

$$14 \text{ stones} = 88.9 \text{ kg}$$
$$4 \text{ pounds} = 1.8 \text{ kg} \quad \text{(add the two together)}$$
$$\overline{90.7} \text{ kg}$$

ANSWER: 91 kg (to nearest kg)

Using the conversion factors

Use the conversion factor: stones to kilograms (multiply by 6.3503)

$$14 \text{ stones} = 14 \times 6.3503 = 88.9042 \text{ kg}$$

Use the conversion factor: pounds to kilograms (multiply by 0.4536)

$$4 \text{ pounds} = 4 \times 0.4536 = 1.8144 \text{ kg}$$

$$14 \text{ stones} = 88.9042 \text{ kg}$$
$$4 \text{ pounds} = 1.8144 \text{ kg} \quad \text{(add the two together)}$$
$$\overline{90.7186} \text{ kg}$$

ANSWER: 91 kg (to nearest kg)

Many parents are more familiar with a baby or child's weight in pounds and ounces. They may ask you to convert from metric to imperial units.

GRAMS TO OUNCES		KILOGRAMS TO POUNDS	
GRAMS	**OUNCES**	**KILOGRAMS**	**POUNDS**
5	0.18	1	2.2
10	0.35	2	4.4
20	0.70	3	6.6
30	1.1	4	8.8
40	1.4	5	11.0
50	1.8	6	13.2
60	2.1	7	15.4
70	2.5	8	17.6
80	2.8	9	19.8
90	3.2	10	22.0
100	3.53		
200	7.05		
300	10.6		
400	14.1		
500	17.6		
600	21.2		
700	24.7		
800	28.2		
900	31.7		

Note: Conversion factors are as follows:

Grams to ounces $\times$ 0.035274

Kilograms to pounds $\times$ 2.2046

Appendix 3

HEIGHT CONVERSION TABLES

Sometimes it may be necessary to convert feet and inches to centimetres and vice versa. Patients' heights are usually given in feet and inches and have to be converted to centimetres. Some dosages are calculated on a 'surface area basis', e.g. mg/m^2, particularly cytotoxic drugs.

The following table shows height conversions.

FEET TO CENTIMETRES		INCHES TO CENTIMETRES	
FEET	**CENTIMETRES**	**INCHES**	**CENTIMETRES**
1	30.5	1	2.5
2	61.0	2	5.1
3	91.4	3	7.6
4	121.9	4	10.2
5	152.4	5	12.7
6	182.9	6	15.2
		7	17.8
		8	20.3
		9	22.9
		10	25.4
		11	27.9

Note: Lengths in centimetres correct to 0.1 cm.

Conversion factors:
Feet to centimetres × 30.48
Inches to centimetres × 2.54
Centimetres to feet × 0.028
Centimetres to inches × 0.3937

WORKED EXAMPLE
Convert 6 feet 2 inches to centimetres (to the nearest cm).

Using the conversion table

$$6 \text{ feet} = 182.9 \text{ cm}$$
$$2 \text{ inches} = \underline{5.1} \text{ cm (add the two together)}$$
$$188.0 \text{ cm}$$

ANSWER: 188 cm (to nearest cm)

Using the conversion factors
Use the conversion factor: feet to centimetres (multiply by 30.48)

$$6 \text{ feet} = 6 \times 30.48 = 182.88 \text{ cm}$$

Use the conversion factor: inches to centimetres (multiply by 2.54)

2 inches = 2 × 2.54 = 5.08 cm
6 feet   = 182.88 cm
2 inches =   5.08 cm (add the two together)
             187.96 cm

ANSWER: 188 cm (to nearest cm)

Appendix 4

CALCULATION OF BODY MASS INDEX (BMI)

Body mass index or BMI (wt/ht^2), based on an individual's height and weight, is a helpful indicator of obesity and underweight in adults.

BMI compares well to body fat but cannot be interpreted as a certain percentage of body fat. The relation between fatness and BMI is influenced by age and gender. For example, women are more likely to have a higher per cent of body fat than men for the same BMI. At the same BMI, older people have more body fat than younger adults.

BMI is used to screen and monitor a population to detect risk of health or nutritional disorders. In an individual, other data must be used to determine if a high BMI is associated with increased risk of disease and death for that person. BMI alone is not diagnostic.

A healthy BMI for adults is between 18.5 and 24.9. BMI ranges are based on the effect body weight has on disease and death. A high BMI is predictive of death from cardiovascular disease. Diabetes, cancer, high blood pressure and osteoarthritis are also common consequences of overweight and obesity in adults. Obesity itself is a strong risk factor for premature death.

BMI GUIDELINES

Underweight	BMI <18.5
Acceptable	BMI 18.5–25
Overweight	BMI 25–30
Obese	BMI 30–40
Morbidly obese	BMI >40

Online calculator

https://www.medicinescomplete.com/mc/bnf/current/PHP18584-body-mass-index.htm

Formula and nomogram

Calculate the BMI for a patient with height = 188 cm and weight = 91 kg.

$$BMI = \frac{weight\ (kg)}{height \times height\ (m^2)}$$

In this case, height = 1.88 m; so, $1.88 \times 1.88 = 3.53$ m^2

$$BMI = \frac{91}{3.53} = 25.7 = 26$$

From the table, a weight of 91 kg and a height of 1.88 m would give a BMI of 26

Table 2		Feet	5	5	5	5	5	5	5	5	5	5	5	5	6	6	6	6	6	6	6	6
		Inches	0	1	2	3	4	5	6	7	8	9	10	11	0	1	2	3	4	5	6
		Metres	1.52	1.55	1.57	1.6	1.63	1.65	1.68	1.7	1.73	1.75	1.78	1.8	1.83	1.85	1.88	1.91	1.93	1.96	1.98
Stones	Pounds	Kilograms																			
14	4	91	39	38	37	36	34	33	32	31	30	30	29	28	27	27	26	25	24	24	23

Table 1

Stones	Pounds	Metres → Kilograms ↓	5'0" 1.52	5'1" 1.55	5'2" 1.57	5'3" 1.60	5'4" 1.63	5'5" 1.65	5'6" 1.68	5'7" 1.70	5'8" 1.73	5'9" 1.75	5'10" 1.78	5'11" 1.80	6'0" 1.83	6'1" 1.85	6'2" 1.88	6'3" 1.91	6'4" 1.93	6'5" 1.96	6'6" 1.98
6	0	38	16	16	15	15	14	14	13	13	13	12	12	12	11	11	11	10	10	10	10
6	2	39	17	16	16	15	15	14	14	13	13	13	12	12	12	11	11	11	10	10	10
6	4	40	17	17	16	16	15	15	14	14	13	13	13	12	12	12	11	11	11	10	10
6	6	41	18	17	17	16	15	15	15	14	14	13	13	13	12	12	12	11	11	11	10
6	8	42	18	17	17	16	16	15	15	15	14	14	13	13	13	12	12	12	11	11	11
6	10	43	19	18	17	17	16	16	15	15	14	14	14	13	13	13	12	12	12	11	11
6	12	44	19	18	18	17	17	16	16	15	15	14	14	14	13	13	12	12	12	11	11
7	0	44	19	18	18	17	17	16	16	15	15	14	14	14	13	13	12	12	12	11	11
7	2	45	19	19	18	18	17	17	16	16	15	15	14	14	13	13	13	12	12	12	11
7	4	46	**20**	19	19	18	17	17	16	16	15	15	15	14	14	13	13	13	12	12	12
7	6	47	**20**	**20**	19	18	18	17	17	16	16	15	15	15	14	14	13	13	13	12	12
7	8	48	**21**	**20**	19	19	18	18	17	17	16	16	15	15	14	14	14	13	13	12	12
7	11	49	**21**	**20**	**20**	19	18	18	17	17	16	16	15	15	15	14	14	13	13	13	13
7	12	50	**22**	**21**	**20**	**20**	19	18	18	17	17	16	16	15	15	15	14	14	13	13	13
8	0	51	**22**	**21**	**21**	**20**	19	19	18	18	17	17	16	16	15	15	14	14	14	13	13
8	2	52	**23**	**22**	**21**	**20**	**20**	19	18	18	17	17	16	16	16	15	15	14	14	14	13
8	4	53	**23**	**22**	**22**	**21**	**20**	19	19	18	18	17	17	16	16	15	15	15	14	14	14
8	6	54	**23**	**22**	**22**	**21**	**20**	**20**	19	19	18	18	17	17	16	16	15	15	15	14	14

Continued

14	14	14	15	15	15	15	16	16	16	16	16	17	17	17	17	18
14	14	15	15	15	15	16	16	16	16	17	17	17	17	17	18	18
14	15	15	15	16	16	16	16	17	17	17	17	17	18	18	18	19
15	15	15	16	16	16	16	17	17	17	18	18	18	18	18	19	19
15	16	16	16	16	17	17	17	18	18	18	18	18	19	19	19	20
16	16	16	17	17	17	18	18	18	18	19	19	19	19	20	20	20
16	16	17	17	17	18	18	18	19	19	19	19	19	20	20	20	21
17	17	17	18	18	18	19	19	19	19	20	20	20	20	21	21	21
17	17	18	18	18	19	19	19	20	20	20	20	21	21	21	21	22
18	18	18	19	19	19	20	20	20	21	21	21	21	22	22	22	23
18	18	19	19	19	20	20	20	21	21	21	21	22	22	22	23	23
19	19	19	20	20	20	21	21	21	22	22	22	22	23	23	24	24
19	19	20	20	21	21	21	22	22	22	23	23	23	23	24	24	24
20	20	21	21	21	22	22	22	23	23	24	24	24	24	25	25	25
20	21	21	21	22	22	23	23	23	24	24	24	24	25	25	26	26
21	21	22	22	23	23	23	24	24	25	25	25	25	26	26	27	27
22	22	23	23	24	24	24	25	25	26	26	26	26	27	27	28	28
22	23	23	24	24	25	25	25	26	26	27	27	27	27	28	28	29
23	24	24	25	25	26	26	26	27	27	28	28	28	29	29	29	30
54	55	56	57	58	59	60	61	62	63	64	64	65	66	67	68	69
8	10	12	0	2	4	6	8	10	12	0	2	4	6	8	10	12
8	8	8	9	9	9	9	9	9	9	10	10	10	10	10	10	10

Key: BMI <18.5 = Underweight; BMI 18.5–25 = Acceptable; BMI 25–30 = Overweight; BMI 30–40 = Obese; BMI >40 = Morbidly obese.

Table 2

Stones	Pounds	Kilograms	6'6" 1.98	6'5" 1.96	6'4" 1.93	6'3" 1.91	6'2" 1.88	6'1" 1.85	6'0" 1.83	5'11" 1.8	5'10" 1.78	5'9" 1.75	5'8" 1.73	5'7" 1.7	5'6" 1.68	5'5" 1.65	5'4" 1.63	5'3" 1.6	5'2" 1.57	5'1" 1.55	5'0" 1.52
11	0	70	18	18	19	19	20	20	21	22	22	23	23	24	25	26	26	27	28	29	30
11	2	71	18	18	19	19	20	21	21	22	22	23	24	25	25	26	27	28	29	30	31
11	4	72	18	19	19	20	20	21	21	22	23	24	24	25	26	26	27	28	29	30	31
11	6	73	19	19	20	20	20	21	22	23	23	24	24	25	26	27	27	29	30	30	32
11	8	73	19	19	20	20	21	21	22	23	23	24	24	25	26	27	27	29	30	30	32
11	10	74	19	19	20	20	21	22	22	23	23	24	25	26	26	27	28	29	30	31	32
11	12	75	19	20	20	21	21	22	22	23	24	24	25	26	27	28	28	29	30	31	32
12	0	76	19	20	20	21	22	22	23	23	24	25	25	26	27	28	29	30	31	32	33
12	2	77	20	20	21	21	22	22	23	24	24	25	26	27	27	28	29	30	31	32	33
12	4	78	20	20	21	21	22	22	23	24	25	25	26	27	28	29	29	30	32	32	34
12	6	79	20	20	21	22	22	23	24	24	25	26	26	27	28	29	30	31	32	33	34
12	8	80	20	21	21	22	23	23	24	25	25	26	27	28	28	29	30	31	32	33	35
12	10	81	21	21	22	22	23	24	24	25	26	26	27	28	29	30	30	32	33	34	35
12	12	82	21	21	22	22	23	24	24	25	26	27	27	28	29	30	31	32	33	34	35
13	0	83	21	22	22	23	23	24	25	26	26	27	28	29	29	30	31	32	34	35	36
13	2	83	21	22	22	23	23	24	25	26	26	27	28	29	29	30	31	32	34	35	36

Continued

Weight (kg)	84	85	86	87	88	89	90	91	92	93	93	94	95	96	97	98	99	100	101
Weight (st-lb)	13-4	13-6	13-8	13-10	13-12	14-0	14-2	14-4	14-6	14-8	14-10	14-12	15-0	15-2	15-4	15-6	15-8	15-10	15-12
	21	22	22	22	22	23	23	23	23	24	24	24	24	24	25	25	25	26	26
	22	22	22	23	23	23	23	24	24	24	24	24	25	25	25	26	26	26	26
	23	23	23	23	24	24	24	24	25	25	25	25	26	26	26	26	27	27	27
	23	23	24	24	24	24	25	25	25	25	25	26	26	26	27	27	27	27	28
	24	24	24	25	25	25	25	26	26	26	26	27	27	27	27	28	28	28	29
	25	25	25	25	26	26	26	27	27	27	27	27	28	28	28	29	29	29	30
	25	25	26	26	26	27	27	27	27	28	28	28	28	29	29	29	30	30	30
	26	26	27	27	27	27	28	28	28	29	29	29	29	30	30	30	31	31	31
	27	27	27	27	28	28	28	29	29	29	29	30	30	30	31	31	31	32	32
	27	28	28	28	29	29	29	30	30	30	30	31	31	31	32	32	32	33	33
	28	28	29	29	29	30	30	30	31	31	31	31	32	32	32	33	33	33	34
	29	29	30	30	30	31	31	31	32	32	32	33	33	33	34	34	34	35	35
	30	30	30	31	31	32	32	32	33	33	33	33	34	34	34	35	35	35	36
	31	31	32	32	32	33	33	33	34	34	34	35	35	35	36	36	36	37	37
	32	32	32	33	33	33	34	34	35	35	35	35	36	36	37	37	37	38	38
	33	33	34	34	34	35	35	36	36	36	36	37	37	38	38	38	39	39	39
	34	34	35	35	36	36	37	37	37	38	38	38	39	39	39	40	40	41	41
	35	35	36	36	37	37	37	38	38	39	39	39	40	40	40	41	41	42	42
	36	37	37	38	38	39	39	39	40	40	40	41	41	42	42	42	43	43	44

Key: BMI <18.5 = Underweight; BMI 18.5–25 = Acceptable; BMI 25–30 = Overweight; BMI 30–40 = Obese; BMI >40 = Morbidly obese.

Table 3

Stones	Pounds																				
		Feet	6	6	6	6	6	6	6	5	5	5	5	5	5	5	5	5	5	5	5
		Inches	6	5	4	3	2	1	0	11	10	9	8	7	6	5	4	3	2	1	0
		Metres	1.98	1.96	1.93	1.91	1.88	1.85	1.83	1.8	1.78	1.75	1.73	1.7	1.68	1.65	1.63	1.6	1.57	1.55	1.52
		Kilograms																			
16	0	102	26	27	27	28	29	30	30	31	32	33	34	35	36	37	38	40	41	42	44
16	2	103	26	27	28	28	29	30	31	32	33	34	34	36	36	38	39	40	42	43	45
16	4	103	26	27	28	28	29	30	31	32	33	34	34	36	36	38	39	40	42	43	45
16	6	104	27	27	28	29	29	30	31	32	33	34	35	36	37	38	39	41	42	43	45
16	8	105	27	27	28	29	30	31	31	32	33	34	35	36	37	39	40	41	43	44	45
16	10	106	27	28	28	29	30	31	32	33	33	35	35	37	38	39	40	41	43	44	46
16	12	107	27	28	29	29	30	31	32	33	34	35	36	37	38	39	40	42	43	45	46
17	0	108	28	28	29	30	31	32	32	33	34	35	36	37	38	40	41	42	44	45	47
17	2	109	28	28	29	30	31	32	33	34	35	36	36	38	39	40	41	43	44	45	47
17	4	110	28	29	29	30	31	32	33	34	35	36	37	38	39	40	41	43	45	46	48
17	6	111	28	29	29	30	31	32	33	34	35	36	37	38	39	41	42	43	45	46	48
17	8	112	29	29	29	31	32	33	33	35	35	37	37	39	40	41	42	44	45	47	48
17	10	112	29	29	30	31	32	33	33	35	35	37	37	39	40	41	42	44	45	47	48
17	13	114	29	29	30	31	32	33	33	35	35	37	37	39	40	42	43	45	46	47	49
18	0	114	29	30	31	31	32	33	34	35	36	37	38	39	40	42	43	45	46	47	49
18	2	115	29	30	31	32	33	34	34	35	36	38	38	40	41	42	43	45	47	48	50
18	4	116	30	30	31	32	33	34	34	36	36	38	39	40	41	43	44	45	47	48	50
18	6	117	30	30	31	32	33	34	35	36	37	38	39	40	41	43	44	46	47	49	51

Continued

Stone	lb	Weight																		
18	8	118	51	49	48	46	44	43	42	41	39	39	37	36	35	34	33	32	32	31	30
18	10	119	52	50	48	46	45	44	42	41	40	39	38	37	36	35	34	33	32	31	30
18	12	120	52	50	49	47	45	44	43	42	40	39	38	37	36	35	34	33	32	31	31
19	0	121	52	50	49	47	46	44	43	42	40	40	38	37	36	35	34	33	32	31	31
19	2	122	53	51	49	48	46	45	43	42	41	40	39	38	36	36	35	33	33	32	31
19	4	122	53	51	49	48	46	45	43	42	41	40	39	38	36	36	35	33	33	32	31
19	6	123	53	51	50	48	46	45	44	43	41	40	39	38	37	36	35	34	33	32	31
19	8	124	54	52	50	48	47	46	44	43	41	40	39	38	37	36	35	34	33	32	32
19	10	125	54	52	51	49	47	46	44	43	42	41	39	39	37	37	35	34	34	33	32
19	12	126	55	52	51	49	47	46	45	44	42	41	40	39	38	37	36	34	34	33	32
20	0	127	55	53	52	50	48	47	45	44	42	41	40	39	38	37	36	35	34	33	33
20	2	128	55	53	52	50	48	47	45	44	42	42	40	39	38	37	36	35	34	33	33
20	4	129	56	54	52	50	49	47	46	45	42	42	41	40	39	38	36	35	34	34	33
20	6	130	56	54	53	51	49	48	46	45	43	42	41	40	39	38	37	36	35	34	33
20	8	131	57	55	53	51	49	48	46	45	43	42	41	40	39	38	37	36	35	34	34
20	10	132	57	55	54	52	50	48	47	46	43	43	42	41	39	39	37	36	35	34	34
20	12	132	57	55	54	52	50	48	47	46	44	43	42	41	39	39	37	36	35	34	34

Key: BMI <18.5 = Underweight; BMI 18.5–25 = Acceptable; BMI 25–30 = Overweight; BMI 30–40 = Obese; BMI >40 = Morbidly obese.

Appendix 5

ESTIMATION OF RENAL FUNCTION

Various formulae have been devised, but two that are most commonly used are:

- Cockcroft and Gault equation
- Modified Diet in Renal Disease (MDRD) equation – commonly known as eGFR (estimated glomerular filtration rate)

Both equations rely on measurement of serum creatinine. Creatinine is a muscle breakdown product and the serum concentration of creatinine will not change from day to day because the rate of production is constant and is equal to the rate at which it is eliminated from the body by the kidneys. Thus creatinine clearance is used as a measure of the glomerular filtration rate (GFR) and hence renal function. Various factors affect serum creatinine and include muscle mass, gender, age, weight and race which need to be taken into account.

One major difference between the two equations is that the MDRD equation predicts GFR to a standard body surface area (BSA) of 1.73 m^2 (i.e. the patient's weight is not needed). For this reason, most hospital pathology laboratories use the MDRD equation as they only need to know the serum creatinine.

The Cockcroft and Gault equation predicts a non-normalized creatinine clearance as it takes into account the patient's weight, i.e. it measures what the kidneys are actually doing.

The estimated glomerular filtration rate (eGFR) values are increasingly being reported by hospital laboratories in place of serum creatinine.

When looking at estimations of renal function, it is important to know which calculation has been used to determine GFR – eGFR can give a lower value. The dosing recommendations for drugs used in renal impairment found in reference books and manufacturer's data sheets have used the Cockcroft and Gault equation. Taking these two facts into account, it is recommended that the Cockcroft and Gault equation should be used when adjusting drug doses to an individual's renal function.

Therefore, we will look at the use of the Cockcroft and Gault equation in more detail.

Cockcroft and Gault suggested the following formula that applies to adults aged 20+:

Males:

$$CrCl \ (mL/min) = \frac{1.23 \times (140 - age) \times weight}{serum \ creatinine \ (mcmol/L)}$$

$$CrCl \ (mL/min) = \frac{(140 - age) \times weight}{serum \ creatinine \ (mg/100 \ mL)}$$

Females:

$$CrCl \ (mL/min) = \frac{1.04 \times (140 - age) \times weight}{serum \ creatinine \ (mcmol/L)}$$

$$CrCl \ (mL/min) = \frac{(140 - age) \times weight}{85 \times serum \ creatinine \ (mg/100 \ mL)}$$

TIP BOX

Ensure that the correct value and units for serum creatinine are used.

MEASURING CREATININE CLEARANCE

WORKED EXAMPLE

Male patient aged 67 years, weight 72 kg, having a serum creatinine of 125 mcmol/L

As the units of the serum creatinine are given in mcmol, we must ensure that the right formula is used:

$$CrCl \ (mL/min) = \frac{1.23 \times (140 - age) \times weight}{serum \ creatinine \ (mcmol/L)}$$

where:

age (years) = 67
weight (kg) = 72
serum creatinine (mcmol/mL) 125

Substitute the figures in the formula:

$$CrCl \ (mL/min) = \frac{1.23 \times (140 - 67) \times 72}{125 \ (mcmol/L)} = 51.7 \ mL/min$$

TIP BOX

In the top line, the sum within the brackets is done first, i.e. (140 − 67), then multiply by 1.23 and then by 72: (140 − 67) = 73, so the sum is 1.23 × 73 × 72 = 6464.88.

Online calculator

https://www.medicinescomplete.com/mc/bnf/current/PHP18586-creatinine-clearance.htm

Appendix 6

ABBREVIATIONS USED IN PRESCRIPTIONS

Although directions should preferably be in English without abbreviation, some Latin abbreviations are still used.

The following is a list of common abbreviations that are commonly used and their Latin derivations. It should be noted that the English version is not an exact translation.

ABBREVIATION	LATIN DERIVATION	ENGLISH MEANING
a.c.	*ante cibum*	before food
alt die	*alterna die*	alternate days
appli	*applicatio*	an application
aurist.	*auristillae*	ear drops
b.d.	*bis die*	twice daily
b.i.d.	*bis in die*	twice a day
c or c̄	*cum*	with
c.c.	*cum cibum*	with food (also cubic centimetre)
crem	*cremor*	a cream
D	*dies*	daily
Elix		elixir
gtt (g)	*guttae*	drops
H	*hors*	hour/at the hour of
h.s.	*hora somni*	at bedtime (lit: at the hour of sleep)
INH		inhaler/to be inhaled
Inj		injection
IM		intramuscular
Irrig	*irrigatio*	irrigation
IV		intravenously
IU		International Units
M	*mane*	morning
m.d.u	*more dictus utendus*	to be used or taken as directed
mist	*mistura*	mixture
mitte		please dispense (lit: send)

Continued

ABBREVIATION	LATIN DERIVATION	ENGLISH MEANING
N	*nocte*	night
NEB		nebules/to be nebulized
O	*omni*	every
oculent (oc)	*oculentum*	eye ointment
o.d. (OD)	*omni die*	every day (daily)
o.m. (ON)	*omni mane*	every morning
o.n. (ON)	*omni nocte*	every night
p.c. (PC)	*post cibum*	after food
p.o. (PO)	*per os*	orally (by mouth)
p.r. (PR)	*per rectum*	rectally
p.r.n. (PRN)	*pro re nata*	occasionally (when required)
p.v. (PV)	*per vagina*	vaginally
Q	*quaque*	each/every
		(e.g. q6h = every 6 hours)
q.i.d. (QID)	*quarter in die*	four times a day
q.d.s. (QDS)	*quater die sumendus*	to be taken four times a day
Rx		'recipe' = take
S		without
Sig	*signa*	let it be labelled
SC		subcutaneous
SL		sublingual
s.o.s.	*si opus sit*	if required
STAT	*statum*	at once
supp *or* suppos	*suppositorium*	a suppository
TDD		total daily dose
t.i.d. (TID)	*ter in die*	three times a day
t.d.s. (TDS)	*ter die sumendus*	to be taken three times a day
TOP		topically
U *or* UN		units
Ung	*unguentum*	an ointment

Note: Some of these abbreviations may differ as they depend upon local convention.

INDEX

Note: page numbers in **bold** refer to figures, page numbers in *italics* refer to information contained in tables.